"A professor's professor, Dr. Mendelsohn brings one of his legendary courses to the world outside of his beloved school. With this book, he extends Theodore Reik's legacy and provides a contemporary psychoanalytic guide to case formulation and treatment planning that is at once practical and magical."

J. Christopher Muran, *Ph.D., Gordon F. Derner School of Psychology, Adelphi University; Mount Sinai Beth Israel Psychotherapy Research Program, Icahn School of Medicine at Mount Sinai; NYU Postdoctoral Program in Psychotherapy and Psychoanalysis, New York University*

"Robert Mendelsohn is a teacher and clinician par excellence, having taught clinical psychology at Adelphi University for five decades. Read this book and learn from a clinician who is a master at formulating the client's problems and showing us how to solve them!"

Jacques Barber, Dean, *Derner School of Psychology, Adelphi University, New York*

I0091842

Case Formulation in Contemporary Psychotherapy

Case Formulation in Contemporary Psychotherapy presents a new approach to case conceptualization and case formulation, making meaning from each clinical case and using every piece of data available.

Robert Mendelsohn explains his core basic principles for case formulation, allowing the clinician to assess a case quickly and accurately. This book includes a discussion of the contributions of transference and countertransference, inducement and enactment, as well as the use of paradigmatic techniques, humor, and language. The processes presented, alongside vignettes illustrating their use, will allow clinicians to decode the meaning of all clinical interaction and to communicate that meaning in a helpful way to students and patients.

Providing a new way to access a full range of conscious and preconscious clinical information, *Case Formulation in Contemporary Psychotherapy* will be essential reading for mental health professionals including psychotherapists and psychodynamic and psychoanalytic clinicians in practice and in training. It will also be of great interest to students of psychotherapy and psychoanalysis.

Robert Mendelsohn (Ph.D., ABPP) is Professor of Psychology and former Dean at the Gordon F. Derner School of Psychology of Adelphi University, USA. He has been teaching psychodynamic psychotherapy to mental health professionals for almost 50 years.

Case Formulation in Contempoprary Psychotherapy

Decoding the Conscious and Preconscious Transactions between Therapist, Patient and Supervisor

Robert Mendelsohn

Routledge
Taylor & Francis Group
LONDON AND NEW YORK

Designed cover image: Marc Harris Miller

First published 2024
by Routledge
4 Park Square, Milton Park, Abingdon, Oxon OX14 4RN

and by Routledge
605 Third Avenue, New York, NY 10158

Routledge is an imprint of the Taylor & Francis Group, an informa business

© 2024 Robert Mendelsohn

British Library Cataloguing-in-Publication Data
A catalogue record for this book is available from the British Library

ISBN: 9781032452159 (hbk)
ISBN: 9781032452166 (pbk)
ISBN: 9781003375944 (ebk)

DOI: 10.4324/9781003375944

Typeset in Times New Roman
by codeMantra

… When One Hears Hoof Beats in the Distance, Its Always Horses – Unless It's Zebras …[1]

This is one version of an American medical slang phrase for arriving at a surprising, often exotic, medical diagnosis when a more commonplace explanation is more likely. It is shorthand for the aphorism coined in the late 1940s by Theodore Woodward professor at the University of Maryland School of Medicine, who instructed his medical interns: "… When you hear hoof beats behind you, don't expect to see a zebra …." While horses are common in Maryland, zebras are relatively rare; logically, one could confidently guess that an animal making hoof beats is probably a horse. By 1960, the aphorism was widely known in medical circles.[2]

We will soon see that this book is about the metaphor presented above: but with a different twist. That is, my premise is that in psychological case formulation, one can sometimes hear hoof beats, assume horses, and find, to great surprise, that what we are observing is a herd of zebras.

Notes

1 Coined in the late 1940s by Dr. Theodore Woodward, a professor at the University of Maryland School of Medicine. Credit link: https://en.wiktionary.org/wiki/when_you_hear_hoofbeats%2C_think_of_horses%2C_not_zebras#Alternative_forms
2 Commencement Exercises (PDF) University of Maryland. June 4, 1938, p. 5. Retrieved 2021-01-31. See: https://archive.hshsl.umaryland.edu/bitstream/handle/10713/3875/1938-1948.pdf

Contents

Foreword

**Case Formulation in Contemporary Psychotherapy:
Decoding the Conscious and Preconscious Transactions
between Therapist, Patient and Supervisor**

> *Magic (noun): an extraordinary power or influence seemingly from a super-
> natural source.*
> *Magician (noun): a person with magical powers; a person with exceptional
> skill in a particular area.*

To fully appreciate the groundbreaking clinical framework described by Dr. Robert
Mendelsohn in *Case Formulation in Contemporary Psychotherapy*, it is helpful to
look more closely at the two definitions above (both from the Oxford Languages
Online Dictionary). In this book's Preface, Dr. Mendelsohn describes some events
from what has become a longstanding tradition in Adelphi University's Derner
School of Psychology. At the close of each spring semester, the doctoral students
perform a series of skits lampooning various members of the faculty. In the particular skit that Bob describes, he is portrayed as having stunning—almost unex-
plainable—insight into the psychological makeup of a patient who has just been
presented by a student in a Case Conference. Based solely on a few minor details,
Bob Mendelsohn is able to generate a nuanced and insightful description of the
patient's underlying dynamics and behavior. The Presenter is impressed, and somewhat mystified, by Dr. Mendelsohn's insight: How could he decipher the key elements of this complex case so quickly, and so effortlessly? As Bob describes the
theme of this particular skit:

> What these students are presenting is a parody of a kind of 'clinical magic.' And
> yet, the parody is a comic exaggeration of what appears to them to be a *magical*
> process that does actually occur in my supervisory seminars - and in many of
> my other clinical encounters.

It is magical indeed, and to fully appreciate the important work discussed in this
remarkable volume, one must understand how the magician performs his magic,

and how in doing so he helps his audience take that first step toward becoming magicians themselves.

As its title suggests, this is a book about case formulation. Case formulation (also called *case conceptualization*) has a long history in psychology and psychiatry; modern case formulation can be traced to Freud's writings, in particular his case studies and essays on therapeutic technique. From its inception, psychodynamic case formulation has been based on the premise that symptoms by themselves provide inadequate information for treatment planning and that effective intervention requires a more nuanced understanding of the patient's personality organization and underlying psychological dynamics (e.g., reality testing, impulse control, introspective capacity, and defense style). Case formulation yields an integrated, holistic understanding of the patient, their history, and their current functioning, enabling the therapist to delineate therapeutic goals, develop an appropriate intervention (or set of interventions), and anticipate the transference, countertransference, resistance, and other patient-therapist dynamics that inevitably arise during psychotherapy.

Which leads to a crucial question—a question that captures well the goal and purpose of this book: How can we teach case formulation most effectively to the next generation of clinicians? Dr. Mendelsohn addresses this question early on when he writes:

> This book is about case formulation; that is, it is more than a book about psychotherapy supervision. My goals are both larger and more ambitious. I will present my own approach to case formulation and treatment planning; an approach that I have developed over nearly 50 years. I will also demonstrate the ways in which my approach differs from ongoing psychotherapy supervision. That is, I will show how my approach is much more helpful and effective in very quickly organizing and directing the complex data of each clinical encounter - from the very beginning of the therapy - to its conclusion.

Bob Mendelsohn's unique approach to organizing the complex data of the clinical encounter leverages a fundamental property of the human mental apparatus: We often know more than we realize about ourselves and other people, but we are not always able to access this preconscious knowledge effectively. Bob Mendelsohn's strategy for accessing preconscious (and unconscious) material parallels that of Freud, who, paradoxically, came to realize that the best way to access unconscious content is not to focus on it effortfully, but to direct one's attention elsewhere so that the material can emerge spontaneously. In Bob's words:

> When we open our minds and allow ourselves access to the unconscious experiences in the clinical encounter, these experiences become more available and we become more aware of clinical data that has been there-in the room-all along.

Hence the magic: Like the performer who pulls a metaphorical rabbit out of a hat, by using Dr. Mendelsohn's approach, the clinician can learn how to pull preconscious wisdom out of thin air. The implications of this method go far beyond clinical supervision. For example, one important correlate of this framework is the recognition that patient and clinician are more alike than is often acknowledged, with parallel intrapsychic dynamics, conflicts, fears, wishes, and resistances. Enactments similar to those exhibited by patients within and outside therapy are displayed by the beginning therapist during supervision and case consultation. And no wonder, the patient's conflicts, impulses, and defenses have been unconsciously communicated to the therapist, who then unconsciously communicates this same material to the supervisor. As the case vignettes that are presented throughout this book illustrate, an important advantage of Bob's approach over more traditional consultation methods is that by identifying these enactments as they occur, the Consultant is modeling effective therapeutic attitude and behavior. In Bob Mendelsohn's model of case consultation, teaching occurs not only through talking but also through doing.

Many of us have seen the 1940 Disney film *Fantasia*, and if so, we likely recall one of the more memorable vignettes from that film, *The Sorcerer's Apprentice*. Based on a 1797 poem by Johann Wolfgang von Goethe ("Der Zauberlehrling"), *The Sorcerer's Apprentice* begins as a wise old sorcerer departs his workshop leaving his young apprentice with a series of tasks to perform. Tired of fetching water one pail at a time, the apprentice casts a spell, enchanting a broom to do the work for him. But there's a problem. The apprentice used magic in which he has not been fully trained. Events soon spin out of control, and the workshop is flooded; the apprentice realizes, to his chagrin, that he cannot stop the process because he does not know the magic required to do so. Just when all seems lost, the sorcerer returns, breaks the spell, and saves the day.

The moral of the story is clear. Our students witness magic like that described by Dr. Robert Mendelsohn, and they say to themselves, someday I want to be able to do that too. Our students are apprentice magicians. But acquiring the kind of expertise that enables one to do 'clinical magic' takes many years—perhaps a lifetime—and it is important to understand this too and to recognize what one does not yet know. Like the sorcerer's apprentice, the overeager student must take time to become proficient in therapeutic technique and be careful not to reach beyond their grasp. Only a master magician should invoke powerful spirits.

Robert F. Bornstein, Ph.D.
Adelphi University

Preface

This book is about case formulation; that is, it is more than a book about psychotherapy supervision. My goals are both larger and more ambitious. In this book,
I first trace the major work done previously on the formulation of the therapeutic
treatment plan in psychodynamic psychotherapy. Theories that include a treatment
plan that moves the work from the initial patient contacts through the working
phase of the therapy to its conclusion will be reviewed. This includes the early
works of Alexander and French (1946), Reich (1949), Reik (1948), Bion (1962),
and Winnicott (1960, 1971), as well as some more recent works, including Billow
and Mendelsohn (1990), which looks at the complex transference/countertransfer-
ence patient/therapist interactions. Following this, I will present my own approach
to case formulation and treatment planning, an approach that I have developed over
nearly 50 years. I will also demonstrate the ways in which my approach *differs
from ongoing psychotherapy supervision.* That is, I will show how my approach
is much more helpful and effective in very quickly organizing and directing the
complex data of each clinical encounter, from the very beginning of the therapy to
its conclusion.

That said, before this ambitious undertaking, I want to present an anecdote that
I hope will enrich our discussion and show the reader where I am going and why
I am going there.

I have taught in the doctoral program in clinical psychology at Adelphi University
for 48 years. There is a long tradition in the program, a tradition that has become
legendary in the history of the program (BTW, our doctoral program is itself legendary—as the program has had an important role in the history of clinical psychology as it is currently practiced in the United States).

To continue, the tradition that I will describe soon had its origins in the 1950s,
under the leadership of the late Dr. Gordon F. Derner, my mentor and friend and the
founder of our doctoral program.

The tradition is as follows: as each doctoral class completes their final (fourth)
year of on-campus residency in the program—and before this cohort leaves for a
one-year full-time internship—in a hospital or other clinical setting, the faculty
throws a party for these departing students. As part of the festivities, the students

roast the faculty by performing a series of skits where they show, in parody format, what they have learned about us during their four years here. Faculty will often comment later that there is a certain irony to all of this: we work hard to train our students to become keen observers of human behavior, and then, they show us what they have learned at our expense!

How does this relate to the substance of this book? This is a reasonable question, and I will answer it now.

There is one common *skit theme* performed by two (or more) students. It is a parody that, in one form or another, has been performed by these doctoral cohorts over a span of many years. It is a parody about me.

Two fourth-year doctoral students are facing each other. They are acting as if they are in an actual clinical case conference. These case conferences occur frequently during the students' four years of in-house training with us (before they leave for their internship); in these meetings, a student presents a clinical case to a faculty member/leader; the cases that they present are currently being supervised by another member of our faculty. In this setting, the student (and the 4/5 other members of the seminar) is able to hear a different point of view (i.e., different from their current faculty mentor), and thus, they may hear another way of understanding their case in this professor's formulation (i.e., his/her understanding) of the treatment.

In a typical skit/parody performed about me over the years, one student is wearing a sign around his/her neck that says something like *Student/Case Presenter*, several other students are wearing signs that say *Student*, while facing the *Student/ Presenter* character is a student wearing a sign that says something like *Bob Mendelsohn*.

Here is their typical (parody) *conversation*:

Bob Mendelsohn:	Please tell us what is the patient's age, race, sex, and gender/preference?
Student:	He's a 39-year-old, white, cis-gendered male.
Bob Mendelsohn:	Did he ever play the bassoon?
Student:	Yes, in high school!
Bob Mendelsohn:	Does he speak Estonian?
Student:	Wow, yes, he studied it with a private tutor!
Bob Mendelsohn:	Does he eat all of his meals alone in his yard, while wearing silly clown costumes?
Student:	OMG…Yes!
Bob Mendelsohn:	Now, let's see how this all fits together so we can formulate a treatment plan for this person. I'm guessing that this man's mother didn't think that his father was interesting enough, so she forced her only son to play a less common musical instrument (the bassoon) and to learn an unusual foreign language (Estonian) so he wouldn't disappoint her, as her husband had done (and, I'm guessing, perhaps also

as her own father had done). But the mother's 'plan' back-
fired; now, this patient lives out his life by being strange
and acting strangely, that is, by having strange eating habits
and rituals! Now, based on this profile, I will describe how
I think one should work with him....

Student: This makes so much sense! How do you do this?

This kind of back and forth continues for a bit longer, while the entire audience laughs (including me) and many also nod and smile along.

Of course, the *parody* is that this scene is quite ridiculous! It is a wildly exaggerated scene, and in actuality, it could never have occurred that I would be able to speculate about any of this in an actual clinical presentation, unless I had some secret/inside information about this (rather unusual) patient and this case. What these students are presenting is a parody of a kind of 'clinical magic.' And yet, the parody is a comic exaggeration of what appears to them to be a *magical* process that does occur in my supervisory seminars and in many of my other clinical encounters.

To demonstrate what I am saying, I will now present three brief, but typical (real-life) clinical examples.

Real-Life Clinical Examples

The first is a vignette from part of a couple's therapy session, and the second and third are examples of student case presentations, all of which will demonstrate how a psychodynamic clinician/teacher/supervisor can perform what appears to be a kind of *clinical magic*.

Excerpt of a Session with a Narcissistic Couple: Martin and Trish—Session 6

Here is an example from a vignette of a couple, therapy session, with a couple that I have diagnosed as a *Narcissistic Couple* (c f Mendelsohn 2017).

Martin and Trish are married, with two young children; they are both in their mid-40s; she is a non-practicing attorney who does most of the family childcare, while he is a physician/general surgeon. As will soon emerge, they consider themselves to be quite successful and they are arrogant about their successful lives, but their relationship is in a bit of trouble.

Trish: "Is your office different? It seems brighter ... brighter colors?"
Martin: "I never noticed the office."
Therapist: "It's brighter here."
Trish: (*to Martin*) "I told you."
Therapist: [I'm suddenly feeling anxious because I was presenting what is called a "confrontation," that is, a comment about how color equals

	mood. However, Trish didn't *get it*. She responded as if I was agreeing with her. I'm thinking about clarifying what I meant, but then I think that I might seem foolish. I now think to myself that I can't afford to seem foolish with this couple].[1]
Martin:	"We have bigger issues to deal with than that. I still want to have a reassurance that you won't have any more contact with X [Trish's recent, brief affair]."
Trish:	"I told you that I wouldn't."
Martin:	"What does *your word* count for?"
Therapist:	"Martin needs a way to no longer feel vulnerable."
Martin:	"I don't feel vulnerable."
Therapist:	"I forgot."
Martin:	(*laughing*) "I meant that if she can reassure me, then I'll put this to rest. After all, I haven't been an angel in this marriage, but it's time for both of us to grow up."
Trish:	"You always set the terms."
Therapist:	"I think that both of you are raising interesting points. I think that Trish's comment about the office's colors was a communication that she is feeling 'brighter' (better) about the marriage, and then, I think that you got competitive with each other, as if I couldn't care for the both of you at the same time."
Martin:	"I told you he was smart."
Trish:	"Yes, you did!"
Therapist:	"Well, you agree about that."

The Magic

With regard to this *magic*, I suggest that what matters most in this little vignette is not whether I (their therapist) am *smart* but that the so-called magic that the students (above) had parodied about me (and that Martin and Trish are portraying) is a simple translation of some latent content to its underlying manifest content (i.e., translating it from therapist to couple).[2]

Student Case Presentations

Here is a second clinical example; this time it is a *Student Case Presentation*. A 29-year-old, Caucasian, cis-gendered male student has agreed to present a therapy case in a clinical case conference that includes the Presenter, five other students, and me. I ask about the age, race, sex, and gender preference of the patient, and the student says:

He's a young Caucasian, male; he's 28.

I then ask a few (more pointed) questions, followed by:

Bob: "Do you think that this person is developmentally delayed—
                          perhaps on the (autism) spectrum?"
Student/Therapist: "I didn't think of that, but yeah, I think that he may actually
                          be on the spectrum."

This student/Presenter is also in his late 20s, that is, 28 or 29 years old. Thus, to me,
the first part of the sentence: "He's young" is a meaningful/but gratuitous remark.
What does it mean?[3]

And here is a third clinical case presentation that I believe will demonstrate in
even more detail the essence of what I do.

The Presenter is a 28-year-old black, cis-gendered, single, female.

Consultant: "…What is the age, race, sex, and gender preference of the patient?"
Presenter: "…The patient is a 23-year-old, Caucasian, cis-gendered, married
                 female…"
Consultant: "What is her level of education?"
Presenter: "The patient is completing her BA degree."
Consultant: "…Who does the patient live with?"
Presenter: "…She is currently living with her husband…"
Consultant: *"…Do you think that the marriage is stable?"*

The Presenter replies that she believes that the marriage is a happy one.

I then ask if the patient is under any emotional pressure, and apropos of this
question, the Presenter replies that the patient has few friends and that she was
traumatized in her early childhood by social anxiety and a mild speech impediment
and stutter.

The Presenter now elaborates further that the patient's husband is *her only friend.*
I now ask if the Presenter is worried that the patient is putting too much pressure on
her husband, and the Presenter replies:

   …I didn't think of that, but her husband had initially wanted to have a large
   family. However, the patient says that the husband has recently seemed more
   reticent about having children…

I suggest that perhaps the husband is starting to feel that he is already 'saddled with
a child' and that the Presenter may be more worried about the patient's marital relationship than she had realized. The Presenter agrees that this is possible and now
associates that she couldn't quite understand why she had wanted to present this
case; she believed that it was going well and that the patient was effectively working through her traumatic experience of the shyness/social anxiety in childhood,

but the Presenter now realizes that she (the Presenter) is probably more concerned about the issue of this patient's marriage and its possible tenuous nature; that is, she is part of an enactment (Levinson, 2005).

I now remind the Presenter of two things that had occurred: when I asked about age, race, sex, and gender preference of the patient, she answered by adding that the patient was married, but I hadn't yet asked about this. Also, the Presenter had an unusual answer to the following question:

Who does the patient live with?

Here was her reply:

…She is *currently* living with her husband…

This is an awkward phrase that suggests transitionally, and I was struck by it; this answer, along with the Presenter's urgency to tell me of the patient's marital status, had caused me to wonder if the patient's marital relationship has become tense, awkward, and even *tenuous*.[4]

As I said above about the other clinical vignettes, at the beginning of each inter-action, I don't have a totally clear or accurate understanding of what: "it's brighter here" or "he's young" or "currently" comment means only a beginning understanding that the Presenter's remark about the patient meant *something*. That is, the remark has alerted me to the psychological fact that the comment meant *something more* than a factual comment about the following:

- This Presenter;
- the patient to be presented;
- their mix/relationship; and
- the very act of this Presenter presenting this person to this group at this time.

The process of unraveling the psychological meaning of all of this and of putting the meaning in the context of a valuable learning experience (a learning process that includes a viable psychological theory of motivation and etiology, a technique, and a theory of technique and the formulation of a preliminary treatment plan for the case) is what I plan to teach you in this book. I will do so by describing a theory of clinical communication that includes both the manifest and latent con-tent of patient/therapist and Consultant/Presenter interactions. I will highlight my points by including vignettes from my many years of being a practicing clinician, a teacher of clinical process, and a clinical supervisor.

I also want to state my belief that the students who parody me are actually accurate about one thing—I am a very accomplished clinician/therapist/supervisor/consultant and *I am not afraid to make educated guesses in the quest to more deeply understand the meaning that is occurring in the therapy.* How did I become this?

Schulman (in Mendelsohn 2022) suggests that writers in psychoanalysis (and I would suggest that this is also true about writers in psychodynamic psychotherapy) haven't successfully incorporated an epistemology of psychoanalytic science into their approaches to psychological understanding. Scientific knowledge in many fields where interpretation plays an important role is not dependent on controlled studies, but rather upon the care with which multiple and redundant checks are applied as the work proceeds. The psychoanalyst recognizes how this error-checking process is so much a part of their daily work.

Do experienced psychoanalysts have a special kind of (magical) expertise? Schulman suggests that studies of expertise in many fields show that the most important difference between experts and those less successful is the extensive detailed knowledge of the experts. This permits the experts to focus on problem solution rather than following set methods. Problem-solving strategies employed by experts tend to be carried out with flexibility. They don't use cognitive methods identifiably different from those used by others, but they demonstrate what Schulman calls a well-stocked mind. It's rare that the exact nature of the expertise can be stated in many fields, such as in psychoanalysis and psychodynamic psychotherapy. The clinical situation, where the psychotherapist has had an extensive and wide exposure to the mind and life of many long-term patients (and, with me, a very wide exposure to so many patient/therapist consultation relationships), constitutes a very special form of expertise about this work, one that is often underestimated and not often studied. Therefore, I will work hard in this book to present how a *well-stocked mind* works in asking the right kind of questions and deciphering and communicating the meaning of a clinical experience to one's supervisee/student.

However, what Schulman does not include in his model is that one way to become an accomplished therapist is to become an accomplished supervisor/teacher of therapists, and the best way to become an accomplished supervisor and teacher is to do a lot of clinical supervision and teaching. That is the way it worked out for me and for many of the over 2,000 plus therapists (primarily psychologists, but also psychiatrists, social workers, clinical nurse specialists, psychoanalysts, and mental health counselors) that I have worked with, and helped to train, since 1974 (as of this writing—that is 48 years)! That said, I believe that I can impart enough wisdom in this book so that one will not need 48 years to do this, a few months should be a fine beginning.

Yet, how does one work with the important issues raised by Schulman regarding psychodynamic *expertise* while at the same time continue to work effectively with the student's/Presenter's fantasy of *Teacher Omnipotence—the magic* that was parodied in the 'skit' that I presented above? In this regard, it is worth noting that these omnipotent fantasies are not always discouraged, and may even be encouraged, by new clinicians/students who are hoping that their teacher/supervisor has all the available truth, the *magic*, to teach them everything that they need to know. Psychodynamic psychotherapy is both confusing and scary, and the hope, for omnipotent expert, is much more welcomed by a beginner than one might think.

An In-Depth Discussion of the Three *Real-Life* Examples of My Magic Presented Above

With all the above in mind, let us return to the three examples of my *magic* that were presented above: the clinical case and the two supervisory ones. I propose that the best way to accomplish all that I have offered so far is to present a comprehensive model of how the clinician/teacher works clearly and cogently, why/how we make the choices that we make, and why/how we choose to ask the questions that we ask. Reality often has a way of making *magic* seem *less magical*.

In other words, how do I teach this so-called magic and how can I demonstrate the essence of what I do?

Let's now look more closely at all three examples presented above: the clinical session and the two case presentations. What do they have in common and how are they different?

Here is an example from what might, at the first view, seem to be a very different kind of clinical setting, a locked ward of a mental hospital with very disturbed hospitalized patients.

Early in my clinical training (in the early 1960s), I once observed a young female receptionist in an all-male, locked ward of a mental hospital. This designation meant that the patients were all quite disturbed. As this young woman (I thought somewhat seductively and rather provocatively) walked from one office to another, passing by many male patients, several of these men would begin to rock back and forth in their chairs, and several times one man fell to the ground and made the sign of the cross. What was he telling her/us by this strange gesture? I intuit from this behavior that he viewed this young woman as a sexual object and that he was making a somewhat bizarre external effort to defend himself against internal sexual longings. Instead of doing all this internally (in his head) or scrupulously washing his hands and body or reading the Scriptures so that he could find a passage to calm himself and thereby remove any dangerous sexual thoughts—this man defended himself externally.

That is, one could say that this hospital patient was metaphorically showing us his conflict, as psychotic people sometimes do, in a series of *enactments* in the environment. What neurotics might do more subtly, this man did openly—and, at the time, early in my training to become a clinical psychologist, one of the comments I had been taught to make to acutely psychotic hospitalized patients was a description of their confusion: 'inside' is 'outside' and 'outside' is 'inside'. In fact, those who write fiction intuitively understand this. For example, Shakespeare's portrayal of Hamlet includes many symbolic gestures that are metaphors for the expiation of unknowable and intolerable feelings, and, as seen in the *Bible*, the washing away of guilt is one of many common symbolic rituals in religious practice.

To continue and further deepen this discussion, you will soon see that in this book, I show that human communication contains aspects of projective identification; such processes are the earliest forms of 'communication' between mother and infant, and thus, they are the origin of all communication for our species

(Mendelsohn 2017). I also suggest that each of us learns these processes, but that as we age into, that is, learn to use verbal communication skills—from infancy to childhood—most of us typically stop paying close attention to what we once 'knew intuitively.' Therefore, if we can re-train ourselves to reverse the process and take seriously all that we are feeling with our student and/or patient, all that they are feeling about us (and in a seminar, all that we are feeling about all the other members of the seminar group), we can help ourselves to more consciously know what we actually already unconsciously knew.

A Bit of My History and This Book

My academic interest in psychodynamic treatment, case formulation, and supervision began in the 1970s when I joined the faculty at the Derner School of Psychology of Adelphi University, working with the late Drs. Donald Milman and Gordon Derner. However, my *exposure* to *psychoanalytic magic* goes much further back to the early 1950s (I was born in 1943), when my mother's younger sister, my Aunt Mildred, would tell me stories about Herr Professor Dr. Sigmund Freud and about Mildred's mentor. Mildred's mentor was one of Freud's students, Dr. Theodore Reik, and he was Aunt Mildred's teacher (he referred to Mildred as his protégée). Reik received a Ph.D. degree in psychology from the University of Vienna in 1912. His dissertation was only the second psychoanalytic dissertation written, coming one year after one penned by Dr. Otto Rank. After receiving his doctorate, Reik devoted several years to studying with Freud. Freud financially supported Reik and his family during this time. Reik was himself psychoanalyzed by another of Freud's early students, Dr. Karl Abraham (2002). Reik's most important book, *Listening with the Third Ear* (1948), describes how psychoanalysts intuitively use their own unconscious minds to decipher the unconscious minds of their patients!

I see myself, and this book, as an attempt to continue Reik's (and my aunt Mildred's) work by developing a theory and technique that extends their brilliant insights into the case formulation process; by detailing how the so-called magical process of decoding the unconscious mind of the patient involves listening more closely to the therapist/Presenter's discussion of the material, as well as to one's own inner processes, and then decoding what the presenting therapist doesn't consciously know- but what –I propose-he/she *does know unconsciously*-and knows at a level that is retrievable once he/she learns *how to let themselves know- it.*

To summarize, I began my doctoral studies in clinical psychology in Massachusetts. In 1969, I earned a Ph.D. in clinical psychology from the University of Massachusetts in Amherst, Massachusetts.[5] In 1970, I returned to New York and began my postgraduate study in psychoanalysis and psychotherapy at Adelphi University. At Adelphi, I completed two postdoctoral training programs: a four-year postgraduate program in *psychoanalysis* and *psychotherapy* and a three-year postgraduate program in *group psychotherapy*, both at the Derner School of

Psychology. While I was a postdoctoral student (in 1974), I also began full-time teaching at Adelphi University in the doctoral program in clinical psychology, and later, I began to teach in the postdoctoral program (now the postgraduate program) in psychoanalysis and psychotherapy.

I have been teaching psychodynamic psychotherapy and psychodynamic supervision/case formulation to bright, talented, and demanding doctoral and other mental health cohorts continuously for 48 years. I have also been fortunate to work in an intellectually supportive environment at the Derner School of Psychology of Adelphi University; to have had coursework and clinical presentations with visiting professors such as Drs. Lewis Aron, Habib Davanloo, Reubin Fine, Bernard Frankel, James Grotstein, Earl Hopper, Masud Kahn, Otto Kernberg, Robert Langs, Donald Meltzer, Stephen Mitchell, Adam Phillips, Peter Sifneos, Harold Searles, Hyman Spotnitz, Vamik Volkan, John Warkentin, Alexander Wolf, and Benjamin Wolstein; and to have had clinical supervision with several excellent supervisors, including Dr. W.R. Bion.[6]

Summary

To sum up, my goal for this book is to teach the reader a new way to access a full range of conscious and preconscious clinical information to aid the student as well as the practicing clinician in case conceptualization and case formulation.

The Child, the Family, and the Outside World. Middlesex: Penguin.

Notes

1 There are several reasons why one would not want to 'feel foolish' with the couple presented above. Of course, no clinician ever wants to at least, accidentally, feel foolish with a patient(s), but with this couple, at this stage of their treatment, that would be a particularly difficult challenge. This is related in part to their psychological dynamics, that is, this kind of couple often relies on the sharing of the defenses of idealization and contempt with each other and, often, with the rest of the world. Thus, as we saw in the vignette, I am now *temporarily* being idealized:

   Martin: *"I told you he was smart."*
   Trish: *"Yes, you did!"*

   BTW, the idealization might change in a minute with this couple; at an early stage of the therapy, it would not be helpful; at a later stage, *it could be helpful*. But this is a discussion for another time and place (Mendelsohn 2017). However, my concern about 'feeling foolish' in the current vignette also speaks to a larger issue. This couple might hear my 'ramblings' and conclude that I'm crazy; ironically, technically speaking, they wouldn't be wrong! In this book, I will attempt to show that the ability to reach deeply into the unconscious of another is the ability to touch the deepest layers of the mind. If one can have access to such places, while also maintaining the critical ego functions of reasoning and intellectualization, then one can become a master clinician. If one has such access, but has no such *space* to put away what one sees, thinks, and feels, then the result will affect dysregulation, splitting, and fragmentation of thinking, that is, such a person would probably be considered insane.

2 The translation of a metaphor is one way to understand and decode the hidden meaning of an enactment, that is, of an act or behavior that occurs in a therapy typically as an attempt to work through a person's traumatic childhood. We will see many of these enactments and their translations throughout this book. The tradition of translating from the manifest meaning to the latent content of a person's comments (i.e., not just translating it within the psychoanalyst's office with his/her patient) goes back to Freud's book, *The Psychopathology of Everyday Life* (1901). In that work, which was originally intended for a popular audience, Freud extended his understanding of the unconscious by using insights he had gained from psychoanalyzing neurotic patients and by applying this method to all human communication. Starting with the observation that neurosis is an unconscious defense against intolerable experience, Freud looked at the so-called normal phenomena—such as slips of the tongue and errors of omission—which had previously been thought to be accidental. In this newer work, what is now commonly called 'Freudian slips' are understood as like what occurs in dreaming and neurotic symptoms, that is, these 'slips,' mistakes, and/or what I've called above 'gratuitous comments' also follow an orderly process where there is blocking (repression) of thoughts and emotion followed by a failure of the repression. However, in these non-neurotic phenomena, the failure of repression is temporary; and the interference with functioning is minor and brief. As I said above, this tradition of translating the manifest into the latent content was further extended, elaborated, and applied to many other kinds of clinical processes by Theodore Reik (1948) in his groundbreaking book, *Listening with the Third Ear.*

3 I call them 'gratuitous remarks,' but in fact, as said right after this, I also say that they are actually 'small gifts.' This is my real point. In this setting, they are gifts that one can use to 'decode' the Presenter's preconscious transactions to emerge; *that is why I wait for the Presenter to continue before I intervene and either ask more questions or make a comment. The transactions always do...even when the Presenter doesn't want them to emerge as we will see below.*

4 This interaction provides me with another opportunity to say that I typically do not initially know what a Presenter's gratuitous comments mean; that said, in this vignette, I did know that the awkward placement of the word *currently* suggested an oddity that one sees in slips of the tongue and parapraxis; it was thus worth exploring. In *The Psychopathology of Everyday Life* (1901) and *Jokes and Their Relation to the Unconscious* (1905), Freud extended his understanding of the unconscious mind. He used the insights that he had gained from the psychoanalysis of neurotic patients. Starting with the observation that neurosis is an unconscious defense against intolerable experience, Freud now looked at a variety of the so-called normal phenomena, such as slips of the tongue, which had previously been thought to be accidental, and jokes, where he demonstrated that joke telling, like dreaming, neurotic symptoms, and *Freudian slips* all follow an orderly process where there is a release, or a blocking (repression), of thoughts and emotion followed by a failure of the repression. However, in these phenomena, the failure of repression is temporary and the interference with the person's functioning is minor and brief. As we have seen, as an extension of Freud/ Reich/Reik/Winnicott/Bion in my own work, I have applied this way of understanding as somewhat odd placements of sentences, words or phrases, and add-ons to sentences in the belief that these unusual words and phrases or unusual placement of words and phrases can provide us with insights into preconscious processes in the Presenter. Further, this deeper understanding of the *Presenter* will ultimately lead us to a deeper understanding of the case that is being presented. In other words, I look not only at what the Presenter says but also at what he/she does not say or what he or she says oddly.

5   My academic interest in Freud began in the 1970s when I joined the faculty at the Derner School of Psychology of Adelphi University, working with the late Drs. Donald Milman and Gordon Derner. However, my *exposure* to psychodynamics and to Freud goes much further back to the early 1950s (I was born in 1943), when my mother's younger sister, Aunt Mildred, would tell me stories about Herr Professor Dr. Sigmund Freud. Mildred heard these stories from Dr. Theodore Reik,[2] her teacher and mentor (he referred to Mildred as his protégée). Reik received a Ph.D. degree in psychology from the University of Vienna in 1912. His dissertation was only the second psychoanalytic dissertation written, coming one year after one penned by Dr. Otto Rank. After receiving his doctorate, Reik devoted several years to studying with Freud. Freud financially supported Reik and his family during this time. Reik was himself psychoanalyzed by another of Freud's early students, Dr. Karl Abraham (2002).[1] Reik's most important book, *Listening with the Third Ear* (1948), describes how psychoanalysts intuitively use their own unconscious minds to decipher the unconscious minds of their patients.

  With Mildred as my academic inspiration, I finished my undergraduate studies in New York (and left my *other career* as a rock and roll musician playing drums in music clubs in New York City, where I had played the drums with several later-to-be-famous rock and roll acts, such as Al Kooper and the singing group, The Ronettes). In 1964, I began my doctoral studies in clinical psychology, and in 1969, I earned a Ph.D. in clinical psychology from the University of Massachusetts in Amherst,[2] and then, I spent a year teaching psychology at Hobart and William Smith Colleges in Geneva, New York. In 1970, I returned to Long Island; for several years, I was a supervising psychologist at the Nassau University Medical Center while pursuing postgraduate study in psychoanalysis at another Long Island institution, Adelphi University.

  At Adelphi, I completed two postdoctoral training programs: a four-year postgraduate program in psychoanalysis and a three-year postgraduate program in group psychotherapy. In 1974, while still a postdoctoral student, I also began teaching introductory courses and supervising/teaching psychotherapy as a professor in Adelphi's clinical psychology doctoral program. In fact, my first psychodynamic psychotherapy teacher (not counting my informal exposure by my Aunt Mildred), before my formal psychoanalytic training, was a brief encounter with the late Gordon F. Derner who would later become a very important person in my professional life! In 1966, while I was a doctoral student in clinical psychology at the University of Massachusetts, Amherst, as well as a psychology extern at a Veterans Administration Hospital near my doctoral program, I was asked by my then-VA psychology supervisor to present a tape recording (at the time, a new and exciting process for clinical presentation) to my supervisor's former teacher/mentor, a Dr. Gordon F. Derner. Derner had been Dr. Norman Tallent's (1991) mentor at Columbia University many years before, but Derner had moved to Long Island and had founded a new and different kind of Ph.D. program for clinical psychology at Adelphi College. I knew a little about Adelphi, as I was from a neighboring area of Long Island, but I certainly didn't know what to expect from this experience. Therefore, I was quite surprised when Dr. Derner showed up! In 1966, all male staff at this hospital were required to wear sport jackets, shirts, and ties. Derner fulfilled that requirement, but it was with a cowboy jacket, a cowboy shirt, and a cowboy tie. He also wore a cowboy hat and cowboy boots, and to round out his outfit, his wrists were adorned with a variety of 'Indigenous Persons' (at the time, we called this 'Indian/Native American') jewelry. Gordon was an impressive figure, with tall, 'crew-cut' hair, and he also had very interesting things to say. As the world spins in interesting ways, five years later when I applied and was accepted to Adelphi's postdoctoral (now postgraduate) program in psychoanalysis and psychotherapy, Derner was the first instructor to teach our cohort. And he remembered me! Further, as the world continues to spin, in 1994, that is, 28 years later, I had the joy to teach Dr. Tallent's son, now Dr. Marc Tallent, who would later go on to graduate from our Derner doctoral program!

6 W.R. Bion was an influential English psychoanalyst, who became the President of the British Psychoanalytical Society from 1962 to 1965. I was very fortunate to be supervised by him over a two-day meeting, for 16 hours, in 1976 (cf Mendelsohn, R. 1978).

References

Alexander, F., & French T. (1946) *Psychoanalytic Therapy*. New York: Ronald Press.

Arnold, K. (2006) The need to express and the compulsion to confess; Reik's theory of symptom-formation. *Psychoanalytic Psychology*, *23*(4), 738–7.

Billow, R., & Mendelsohn, R. (1987) The peer supervisory group of psychoanalytic therapists. *Group*, *11*(1), 31–34.

Billow, R. M., & Mendelsohn, R. (1990) The interviewer's presenting problem in the initial interview. *Bulletin of the Menninger Clinic*, *54*(3), 391–414.

Bion, W. R. (1961) *Experiences in Groups*. London: Tavistock Publications.Bion, W. R. (1962) *Learning from Experience*. London: Tavistock.

Bion, W. (1977) Cf, Personal Communication. In R. Mendelsohn (Ed.), Critical factors in short-term psychotherapy. *Bulletin of the Menninger Clinic*, 1978, *42*(2), 133–149.

Freud, S. (1918) From the history of an infantile neurosis. *The Standard Edition of the Complete Psychological Works of Sigmund Freud*, Volume XVII, 7–22.

Levenson, E. (2005) *The Fallacy of Understanding and the Anatomy of Change*. London: Routledge.Mendelsohn, R. (1978) Critical factors in short-term psychotherapy: a summary. *Bulletin of the Menninger Clinic*, 42, 133–148. [This article includes a case supervised by W.R. Bion in 1976]

Mendelsohn, R. (2017) *A Three-Factor Model of Couples Therapy*. Lantham, MD: Lexington Books/Rowman & Littlefield.

Mendelsohn, R. (2022) *Freudian Thought for the Contemporary Reader*. London: Routledge.

Reich, W. (1949) *Character Analysis*. New York: Noonday Press.

Reik, T. (1948) *Listening with the Third Ear*. New York: Grove Press.

Winnicott, D. W. (1960). *The Maturational Processes and the Facilitating Environment*. New York: International Universities Press.

Winnicott, D. W. (1971) *Playing and Reality*. London: Tavistock.

Acknowledgments

I want to thank Marc Harris Miller for this book's cover image. I am fortunate to work in an intellectually supportive environment at the Derner School of Psychology at Adelphi University; to have been mentored by the late Drs. Gordon Derner and Donald Milman; and to work with psychoanalytic/psychodynamic scholars such as Drs. Jacques Barber, Robert Bornstein, Laura Brumariu, Wilma Bucci, Morris Eagle, Jairo Feurtes, Jerold Gold, Mark Hilsenroth, Karen Lombardi, Christopher Muran, Joseph Newirth, Michael O'Loughlin, George Stricker, Kirkland Vaughns, and Joel Weinberger.

I especially wish to thank Drs. Jacques Barber, Dean; Chris Muran, Associate Dean; and Laura Brumariu, Director of Clinical Training, who urged and encouraged me to undertake this project.

Drs. Jacques Barber, Chris Muran, and Robert Bornstein have been generous in every way in offering both editorial and much-needed theoretical/scientific advice, and many of their suggestions have been incorporated into this book. Also, as a respected friend and colleague, over many decades, Dr. Richard Billow and I have shared common training experiences, including the work with Drs. Bernard Frankel, Murray List, W.R. Bion, and Otto Kernberg.

I also want to thank the students who have enriched my professional life and allowed me to be a part of theirs as they learned to become psychology scholars and clinical practitioners. Each of you has touched me and I have learned so much from you over the many years that I have been teaching and supervising your clinical work. To all of you and to the hundreds of students who have taken my case formulation seminar as well as my other clinical seminars over the decades—including the class that just completed their courses with me in May 2022—I thank you all for giving me this most wonderful opportunity.

Finally, I want to share with you my answer to the following question: What is a family?

A family is a group of people who support each member through the cycle of life. My family has been a support to me over many years. Our family contains people from the ages of five (my granddaughter Juliet) to 80 (me), and they include Elise Mendelsohn; Dr. Chelsey Miller; my son-in-law Marc Harris Miller; Tyler Mendelsohn; my precious grandchildren Stella Rose Miller and, the aforementioned, Juliet Lennon Miller; and finally, the love of my life, Dr. Robin Mendelsohn, my sidekick, my companion, my cheerleader, my wife.

About the Author

Robert Mendelsohn (Ph.D., ABPP) is Professor of Clinical Psychology and former Dean at the Gordon F. Derner School of Psychology of Adelphi University in Garden City, New York, USA. He has been teaching psychodynamic psychotherapy to mental health professionals for almost 50 years, and he is the author of over 25 scholarly articles and three books, given as follows:

Mendelsohn, R. (2017) *A Three-Factor Model of Couple Therapy*. Lanham, MD: Lexington Books/Rowman & Littlefield.

Mendelsohn, R. (2022) *Freudian Thought for the Contemporary Clinician: A Primer on Psychoanalytic Theory*. London: Routledge.

Mendelsohn, R. (2023) *Case Formulation and Treatment Planning in Contemporary Psychotherapy: Decoding the Conscious and Preconscious Transactions between Therapist, Patient and Supervisor*. London: Routledge.

Introduction

Why a new book about Case Formulation in psychotherapy? Several books discuss this topic directly; for example, there are the classic texts by Alexander and French (1946) and by Ekstein and Wallerstein (1972) and the more recent works of McWilliams (1999) and Eells (2007). Several other books discuss this topic indirectly; for example, Frawley-O'Dea, M.G. and Sarnat, J.G. (2001) or Rock (1997) in their excellent discussion of psychotherapy supervision. So, why do I want to write a book about Case Formulation? One answer for this is related to my next question: How is Case Formulation the same as and in what ways is it different from Clinical Supervision?

Clinical Supervision and Case Formulation are two of the most basic training components to become a mental health professional. The major difference between Case Formulation and Clinical Case Supervision is that the goal of Case Formulation is *long-term treatment planning*, and therefore, one needs to create a long-term overview of the clinical case, with an understanding of the case's long-term goals, as well as a plan for how one might accomplish these goals. However, in contrast to this, clinical supervision have as its focus the day-by-day/minute-by-minute interactions of a particular session or a few sessions, with only an occasional view/review/overview of the long-term planning of the case and, even less frequently, a formulation of the long-term treatment goal(s) of the case. In fact, the current books devoted exclusively to case formulation are T. Eells' (2007) *Case Formulation in Psychotherapy*—while it is well written and helpful in a general way for the beginning clinician, it does not have a psychodynamic focus—and McWilliams' *Psychoanalytic Case Formulation*—while it does focus on the long-term treatment planning of the psychoanalytic case, it has a very different focus from this book, as you will soon see below. Thus, one's choices are limited; you can look at the dated-classic texts listed above or read the current books on Psychodynamic Therapy Supervision and Formulation and find the pearls of wisdom that can be found in these works—none of which deal directly with the important topic that I will be presenting in this book. This is the dilemma I faced when I began to teach case formulation to my advanced doctoral and postdoctoral students. I have now decided to remedy this by writing what I believe will be a valuable book about this underrepresented, but very important topic.

DOI: 10.4324/9781003375944-1

Relatedly, as we saw parodied above in the Student Skit, there is a question to be asked: Why is Case Formulation, when it is done by an expert who is currently not familiar with the case, *sometimes more accurate* than when it is done by the clinician currently treating the patient and/or by the supervisor who was currently supervising the case?

You have already heard one explanation: that the Consulting Clinician is able *to perform magic*. While there are certainly narcissistic satisfactions attached to this explanation, particularly when I am the person being called *the magician*, the fact is that there are some basic principles that one can follow to be able to know as much as or, at the time of a presentation, perhaps even more than the person who is presenting the case.

Here are some reasons why this is so:

> In a very thoughtful book (a book that helped changed the course of psychoanalytic therapy) Alexander and French (1946) point out that in the earliest (initial) interview with one's patient, the clinician can be compared to a traveler standing on top of a hill overlooking the countryside over which he or she will soon be traveling. At this time, it may be possible for this traveler to see the whole anticipated journey in perspective. However, once he or she has descended into the valley, their perspective needs to be retained in memory *or else it will vanish*. Now, the traveler will be able to examine small parts of the current landscape in much more detail than was possible when viewing from a distance- but the broad relations will no longer be so clear.

In this regard, one can see that a skilled newcomer to the case, a newcomer who currently hears the data, may be in some ways, at least *temporarily*, in a better position to understand the case dynamics than the person who is currently immersed in the many details of the case or even than the current supervisor who may also be similarly immersed. I will return to this point later, but I want to emphasize that the so-called outsider to the case now has the *seemingly magical* perspective that the Presenter may have had some version of earlier in the work!

Yet, having some greater understanding of the case material, a formulation of the patient's basic problems and an overview of how to get from this formulation to a clear plan for the treatment is more than simply having a fresh and new perspective on the existing (conscious) data. If this were the only thing one needed to do, our work here would be done. However, there is more that I am going to teach you. What I will present is not *magic*, it is about delving into some new territory for many who do talk therapy; it is about an understanding and appreciation for what I call the *preconscious transactions* between the therapist, patient and therapy supervisor. I suggest that learning how to do this will often reveal aspects of the case that are not (yet) consciously available to the clinician or his/her teacher *but can be quickly learned and easily applied.* Further, having a fresh perspective can help lead to uncovering the presence of *enactments* in the therapy. That said, it is important to state that I am not the first person to have approached this topic in this way, and I owe a debt of gratitude to those psychoanalyst/psychodynamic psychotherapists who have worked within the paradigm of the *mutual enactments* that occur within the clinician and his/her patient. Most notably, here is the work of Levenson (2005). For Levenson, it is impossible not to interact with the patient, and the therapeutic power of psychoanalytic therapy is derived from the clinician's ability to step back from interactive embroilment, the mutual enactment, and to reflect with the patient on what enactments to which it led. That is, to reflect with the patient on what each was doing to, and with, the other. Invariably, Levenson found, the therapist/patient interaction is a recreation of patterns of experience that typified the patient's early family relationships. Further, since the Consultant and Presenter are not in the room with the patient during the clinical presentation, their dyad is operating at a more removed level of abstraction. This can enable them to see things that the clinician/Presenter alone cannot see during the session.

Further, Theodore Reik (1948, 1959b,c) reminds us that in a famous passage of "A Fragment of an Analysis of a Case of Hysteria-The Case of Dora," Freud (1905) wrote the following:

> …He that has eyes to see and ears to hear may convince himself that no mortal can keep a secret. If his lips are silent, he chatters with his fingertips; betrayal oozes out of him at every pore…
>
> (1905/1953, pp. 77–78).

Freud is here alluding to the inability of mortals to keep their unconscious secrets from others, a thesis that supports the scientific and clinical edifice of psychoanalysis (Reik 1925/1959a,b,c, p. 187).

We will soon begin to look at examples such as the ones presented in the *Preface*—the clinical session and the supervisory ones. We will see that the clinician can learn to perceive and decode those bits of clinical data that 'ooze out of every pore,' and to expand on this metaphor, we will learn how to *soak up this ooze* (these data) *the way a sponge soaks up water*.

But first, in the next section, I will explore the question: What does each of these roles/jobs (one-time-only Consultant versus ongoing teacher/supervisor) have in common/how is each of them different from the other?

What Are the Differences between the Supervisor's Ongoing Relationship versus the Consultant's More Time-Limited Relationship to the Presenting Clinician?

In order to answer this question, I believe that it is important to get a historical perspective to see more clearly how psychoanalytic clinicians have conceptualized the differences between an ongoing clinical supervision that, just as an ongoing therapy, needs to be immersed in the week-to-week details of the patient's life, as well as immersed in the patient/clinician's interactions, versus the one-time-only Consultant's quick view (*overview*) of a continuing psychotherapy case.

Previous Clinicians and Their Approaches to Case Formulation and Treatment Planning: An Overview of What Is to Follow

Even those psychoanalytic therapists who have treated patients two or three times per week over a long period of time recognize that one must formulate a plan for the treatment in the very early sessions. While this plan is by nature always going to have to be flexible and altered with new information, these clinicians have always understood that it is best to have some general schema as opposed to simply following a patient wherever he or she leads us.

Yet, all patients who enter therapy are not the same. Even with neurotic patients, one must be sensitive to closeness and silence with someone who is on the neurotic end but has schizoid dynamics; one needs to remain alert to affect with an obsessive-compulsive patient; and one needs to be particularly careful with boundary issues and triangulation concerns with patients with hysterical features.

With these rules in mind, what is 'formulating' a treatment plan? It is the generating of psychodynamic hypotheses, having them tested, confirmed, and/or disconfirmed. In this regard, it is helpful if we divide any psychotherapy treatment into two phases:

1 A psychodynamic formulation, that is, what triggered the current conflict (and how does the current conflict have its roots in the person's history)?
2 The ongoing psychotherapy treatment

Previous Attempts to Formulate the Treatment Plan in Psychodynamic Therapy

Freud (1918) offered us the first psychodynamic formulation of clinical cases. Freud also introduced a very important psychodynamic technique: 'talk therapy.' This technique is comprised of the following:

1 Free association: The patient is encouraged to say everything that is in his/her mind without editing/revising.
2 Detailed inquiry: The therapist pursues various lines of inquiry that highlight a path to reconstruction.
3 Reconstruction: The therapist helps the patient to connect what happened in his/her childhood to one's current life conflicts.
4 Interpretation: The therapist correlates the patient's reconstructions to his or her current symptoms and character problems which leads to relief from these symptoms and an alteration of the character problems.

From Wilhelm Reich (1949), we will see an emphasis not only on what a patient *does and says* but also on what *is not done and not said.* This gives us many clues to the patient's hidden resistances. Reich suggested that Freud's idea of the basic rule of free association was fine in theory, but that in practice, it is not always easy to follow. In this regard, Reich described what he called latent negative resistance. These latent resistances are often missed, and when they are uncovered, our entire understanding of the case formulation may change.

From Theodore Reik (1957), we will see that repression is a repetition of childhood ruptures in communication. Repressed expressions return as composites of the urge to express one's important objects as well as internalized prohibitions against these expressions. The internalized social anxieties linked to the person's superego both inhibit free expression and produce a need for punishment. Neurotic symptoms are *confessions* that combine unconscious expression with self-punishment. Reik's ideas, in particular, have influenced me to develop a technique of Clinical Consultation that often results in the Presenter *wanting to believe* that what I do is *magical*, that is, I have often uncovered certain *truths* about the case that the Presenter was only vaguely aware of. In this book, I will demonstrate that the belief that I am *magical* is emotionally easier for many presenters than to believe that the techniques I perform are both teachable and learnable; in other words, it is easier to believe that I can perform *magic* than to believe that any clinician can learn the same *magic* and therefore can learn to be, in this poetic sense, *omnipotent*. I will also demonstrate that when we want to make meaning out of each clinical case, we can and should use every bit of data that emerges. In this regard, the group setting is the best place to see this via the interchanges that, as we will soon see, take place among the members.

From Billow and Mendelsohn (1990), we will soon hear about peer supervision groups, *The Peer Supervisory Group for Psychoanalytic Therapists* (1987, 1990) in its various forms, and about how peer supervision is different from ongoing clinical supervision by one's supervisor. In this setting, we will see that there are times when a Presenter can hear from his/her peers or a Consultant better than he/she can hear from a 'supervisor/superior in ongoing clinical supervision.' Under such circumstances, the group and Consultant may be able to provide a context for the Presenter that ongoing supervision cannot provide.

In this quick review, I have summarized some of the authors that we will soon discuss to see how their ideas have directed me toward the new methods that I have developed in case formulation and treatment planning.

The Format of My Case Presentations Is Probably Unlike Any Other You Have Ever Seen

Throughout this book, you will see case presentations where the Presenter answers the most important (and frequently asked) demographic questions, but the Presenter is discouraged from any discussion of the patient's stated *presenting problem*. During the several decades that I have successfully switched to this newer method of case formulation, I have observed many clinicians, even clinicians that have presented case material to me previously, struggle with this new way of working. It is as if for many, there is a pressing need to present a *pre-packaged presenting problem*. In this regard, an early sensory/cognitive psychologist studied perception and described a phenomenon named after her. The Russian psychologist Bluma Zeigarnik (Koffka 1935) postulated a phenomenon called 'The Zeigarnik Effect.' This phenomenon occurs when an activity that has been interrupted may be more readily recalled than one that has not. It postulates that people remember unfinished or interrupted tasks better than completed tasks. In Gestalt psychology, the Zeigarnik effect has been used to demonstrate the general presence of Gestalt phenomenon: not just appear as perceptual effects but also present in cognition.

Yet, here is an obvious question: why do I insist on structuring my case formulations this new way? And why do I also insist on hearing only about the patient's demographics?

This question about demographics is simple to answer: demographics (age, sex, race, gender preference, level of education, etc.) are facts, and these 'facts' generate hypotheses; but then, why no 'presenting problem?' In a word, that is because a presenting problem is a *conclusion,* and thus, it is not a fact; a conclusion may interrupt the generation of *new* hypotheses, and therefore, it can even decrease curiosity!

From my perusal of the literature, mine is a revolutionary approach, and I alert those clinicians who have not done this before to be aware of the inner pulls within you to *solve a clinical problem in advance of studying it by generating a 'presenting problem' for a case that explains the person's problems and therefore puts a lid on attempting to see if more can be learned and understood.*

In this regard, on the front page of this book, I quote a famous physician and his discussion of case formulation in medicine:

> …When One Hears Hoof Beats in the Distance, Its Always Horses---Unless It's Zebras…*

* This is one version of an American medical slang for arriving at a surprising, often exotic, medical diagnosis when a more commonplace explanation is more likely. It is shorthand for the aphorism coined in the late 1940s by Theodore Woodward, a professor at the University of Maryland School of Medicine, who instructed his medical interns: "When you hear hoof beats behind you, don't expect to see a zebra." Since horses are common in Maryland while zebras are relatively rare, logically one could confidently guess that an animal making hoof beats is probably a horse. By 1960, the aphorism was widely known in medical circles.
(From *Commencement Exercises (PDF) University of Maryland. June 4, 1938. p. 5. Retrieved 2021-01-31)*

Here is the reason that I have presented the above quote: there are times when we may be *wrong* in our initial assumptions; that is, we may be wrong when we assume that hoof beats *always equal* horses. I contend that that are times in a case presentation that the presenting problem, as the patient presents his/her complaint and as the therapist/Presenter accepts this complaint as the most important dynamic issue in the therapy, is *not* how one should best understand this patient. That is, there are times when other, perhaps more subtle, issues are the most important issues to consider in the formulation of the treatment.

In sum, I will soon review in depth the work of a number of clinicians that provide us with the historical background for the new model that I will be describing; each of these authors has led me, indirectly through their writings, to what I plan to teach you in this book, and one of them, W.R. Bion, taught me to do this directly (Mendelsohn, R. 1978) by supervising several cases for me and formulating the treatment plan with these cases. Thus, I have been fortunate to have a direct experience (Bion 1977) and an indirect one (Theodore Reik, 1950–1960), both of which influenced my thinking quite early in my personal life as well as in my clinical work. This may help the reader to understand an important question that I have been exploring for several years; *how should one teach psychodynamic expertise?* In this regard, I have struggled with a related issue: how does the teacher both avoid the seduction of believing in his/her own omnipotence and at the same time be able to recognize that the role of an effective teacher is to *possess expertise, acknowledge it to oneself, communicate it clearly, and teach this expertise to others.*

To return to the original premise of this book, given what you have already read about me above, the reader might ask the following question: Do I think that I can perform *magic?*

My answer is No!

But then, what about my reputation; is it true that as has been said about me by hundreds of students for decades:

You tell him 3 bits of information and he will tell you about the whole case.

This is essentially true. So, isn't *that* magic?

Not exactly! What I do believe you will see throughout this book is that the processes that I look at are both different than what you have heard/seen/experienced before in the case presentation format and that they are very powerful. Further, I suggest that these processes can be taught. And, particularly for newer clinicians, these techniques and the ways of thinking connected to them will be extremely helpful in decoding the meaning of all clinical interaction and communicating that meaning in a helpful way to one's students and patients. I also believe that these techniques will result in altering the symptoms and character issues of the patients. And, finally, I believe that my procedures will prepare one to become an expert clinician and an expert supervisor/teacher. I recognize that I am promising a lot.

A Further Word about Teacher Omnipotence and My Clinical Vignettes

As I will do throughout this book, I now want to say a bit more about the complex issues going on within the *expert.* I suggest that an expert must struggle with not denying the special skills and power of a supervisor/teacher, yet at the same time learn how to not encourage fantasies of omnipotence within the student. In this regard, in this book, I will teach you ways to look closely at the supervisees' fantasy of 'supervisor omnipotence'—this is the so-called magic that was parodied in the 'skit' presented above.

Let's now look at this fantasy more closely: I suggest that omnipotent fantasies about the clinician/teacher are often not discouraged by one's students and that these students may even subtly encourage these fantasies (sometimes the supervisor encourages them, as well). At some level, beginning clinicians are hoping that their teacher/supervisor has all of the truth, the *magic*, to teach them as clinical work can be both confusing and scary. And, of course, sometimes the supervisor will feel this also perhaps for similar reasons.

However, one thing I hope to communicate in this book is the following: if the supervisor/teacher can begin to recognize and understand the pushes and pulls inside of himself or herself to be omnipotent, and the seductive pushes and pulls that are also coming from their students, and indirectly via preconscious enactments, from the Presenter's patient, this can allow the Consultant to create a space between all of the pushes and pulls within. An awareness of such processes, as well as one's own rational desire to utilize our well-stocked mind, that is, our expertise, can protect the Consultant from not being pulled into enactments in the same way that the Presenter may have been pulled into them. What we will then have instead is a well-earned expertise living side by side, with our own humility, fallibility, curiosity, and, ultimately, with our own awe about the human condition in all its complexity. Further, having a fresh perspective can help lead to the uncovering of *enactments* in the therapy. It is important to state that I am not the first person to have approached this topic in this way, and I owe a debt of gratitude to those psychoanalyst/psychodynamic psychotherapists who have worked within the paradigm of the *mutual enactments* that occur within the clinician and his/her patient. As I have said above, most notably here is the work of Levenson (2005). For Levenson, it is impossible not to interact with the patient, and the therapeutic power of psychoanalytic therapy is derived from the clinician's ability to step back from interactive embroilment, the mutual enactment, and to reflect with the patient on what enactments to which it led, that is, to reflect with the patient on what each was doing to, and with, the other. Invariably, Levenson found that the therapist/patient interaction is a recreation of patterns of experience that typified the patient's early family relationships. Further, since the Consultant and Presenter are not in the room with the patient during the clinical presentation, their dyad is operating at a more removed level of abstraction. This can enable them to see things that the clinician/Presenter alone cannot see during the session.

To summarize, I propose that the best way to accomplish all that I have offered above is to clearly and cogently present a comprehensive model of how the clinician/teacher thinks about his/her cases and how he/she thinks about the best way to perform their work (in other words, the why and how we make the choices and decisions that we make; the why and how we ask the questions that we ask; and the why and how we come to the formulations that we arrive at). Reality has a way of making *magic* seem *less magical.*

Some Words about Format

This book presents a revised model of psychodynamic case formulation that encourages exploring the preconscious transactions as well as the dynamics of the teacher/student from the exact moment of initial presentation (including the first few words spoken) about the 'case.' Why then? This book will also explain this to you in great depth as we go on.

Examples of this case formulation process come from many hours of teaching and supervision over five years (2018–2022). The examples/excerpts of actual teaching interactions have been recorded, transcribed, edited, and then integrated so that they maintain sequence and rhythm. They are included to demonstrate that while the parody of an 'example' of my ork in the skit presented above is silly and exaggerated, like all parodies—there is a certain grain of truth in the example in that—while what I do might sometimes appear to seem like magic, what is occurring is that as the clinical Consultant, I am simply following all of the threads of the therapist/Presenter as he/she presents their actual clinical interaction in the session to be supervised.

In this regard, in all of the examples presented in this book, the identity of both the therapist/Presenter and the patient (or patient(s)—the couple, family, or therapy group) have been disguised—and the data about all members of this clinical encounter (except for me) have been altered to preserve anonymity—while not altering the essential elements of the dynamics, defensive structure, transference-countertransference, unconscious object relations, and preconscious transactions of the experience.

To Summarize

The above is my answer to the question: Do I perform/teach *magic* and can I demonstrate the 'it' of what I do so that it becomes both less magical and more doable? To repeat: I (simply) follow the principles that I have developed and teach what I have learned about the therapist/patient duo in each clinical encounter while also demonstrating *how it is that I have arrived at my conclusion(s).*

References

Alexander, F., & French, T. (1946) *Psychoanalytic Therapy*. New York: Ronald Press.

Billow, R., & Mendelsohn, R. (1987) The peer supervisory group of psychoanalytic therapists. *Group, 11*(1), 31–46.

Billow, R. M., & Mendelsohn, R. (1990) The interviewer's presenting problem in the initial interview. *Bulletin of the Menninger Clinic, 54*(3), 391–414.Eells, T. (2007) *Case Formulation in Psychotherapy.*Washington, DC: American Psychological Association.

Ekstein, R., & Wallerstein, R. S. (1972) *The Teaching and Learning of Psychotherapy*, 2nd edition. New York: International Universities Press.

Frawley-O'Dea, M. G., & Sarnat, J. E. (2001) *The Supervisory Relationship: A Contemporary Psychodynamic Approach*. Guilford Press (Dr. Frawley O'Dea is a graduate of our doctoral program).

Freud, S. (1905) Fragment of an analysis of a case of hysteria. In *The Standard Edition of the Complete Psychological Works of Sigmund Freud, Volume VII* (pp. 3–122).

Freud, S. (1918) From the history of an infantile neurosis. In J. Strachey et al. (Trans.), *The Standard Edition of the Complete Psychological Works of Sigmund Freud, Volume XVII ("Wolf Man")* (pp. 7–122). London: Hogarth.

Freud, S. (1953) Fragment of an analysis of a case of hysteria. In J. Strachey (Ed. & Trans.), *The Standard Edition of the Complete Psychological Works of Sigmund Freud*.

Freud, S. (1955) Group psychology and the analysis of the ego. In J. Strachey (Ed. & Trans.), *The Standard Edition of the Complete Psychological Works of Sigmund Freud* (Vol. 18, pp. 69–143). London: Hogarth Press (Original work published 1921).

Freud, S. (1957) Mourning and melancholia. In J. Strachey (Ed. & Trans.), *The Standard Edition of the Complete Psychological Works of Sigmund Freud* (Vol. 14, pp. 237–258). London: Hogarth Press (Original work published 1917).

Koffka, K. (1935) *Principles of Gestalt Psychology* (p. 334). New York: Keegan, Paul Trubner and co.

Levenson, E. (2005) *The Fallacy of Understanding and The Anatomy of Change*. London: Routledge.

McWilliams, N. (1999) *Psychoanalytic Case Formulation*. New York: Guilford Press.

Mendelsohn, R. (1978) "Critical factors in short-term psychotherapy: A summary. *Bulletin of the Menninger Clinic, 42*(2), 133–148.

Reich, W. (1949) *Character Analysis*. New York: Noonday Press.

Reik, T. (1948) *Listening with the Third Ear: The Inner Experience of a Psychoanalyst*. New York: Grove Press.

Reik, T. (1957) *Myth and Guilt: The Crime and Punishment of Mankind*. New York: George Braziller, Inc.

Reik, T. (1959a) About the genesis of the superego. In J. Farrar (Ed.), *The Compulsion to Confess and the Need for Punishment* (pp. 462–467). New York: Farrar, Straus, and Cudahy.

Reik, T. (1959b) The compulsion to confess. In J. Farrar (Ed.), *The Compulsion to Confess and the Need for Punishment* (pp. 176–356). New York: Farrar, Straus, and Cudahy (Original work published 1925).

Reik, T. (1959c) The unknown murderer. In J. Farrar (Ed.), *The Compulsion to Confess and the Need for Punishment* (pp. 3–173). New York: Farrar, Straus, and Cudahy (Original work published 1932).

Rock, M. H. (Ed.) (1997) *Psychodynamic Supervision: Perspectives of the Supervisor and the Supervisee* (M. H. Rock, Ed.). Northvale, NJ: Jason Aronson.

Chapter 1

The History of Case Formulation and Treatment Planning

From Freud (1918) to W. Reich (1946); from Reich to T. Reik (1948, 1959); from Reik to Bion (1962, 1976) and Winnicott (1960, 1971) to Billow and Mendelsohn (1990)

Sigmund Freud (1918)

Sigmund Freud provided the first model for the presentation of psychoanalytic case formulation via the case history format. Freud's initial work was with Josef Breuer and was published in *Studies on Hysteria* (1895). This was also Freud's first major written work, and it marks the beginning of what later would become psychoanalysis.

This work and all that followed revolve around the observation that neurosis is a psychological defense against intolerable experiences. Freud suggested that the neurotic suffers a trauma and represses (forcefully forgets) traumatic experiences. However, these traumatic thoughts and feelings can break through the repression and become converted into anxiety, psychological symptoms, and/or inhibitions. Freud originally used the hypnotic method that he'd learned from his studies with Charcot,[1] but he soon abandoned it. He did so for two reasons. Freud found the results obtained from hypnosis to be unreliable. Relatedly, he began to suspect that the heightened state of suggestibility associated with hypnosis raises the risk that any repressed memories recovered during the hypnosis might be false memories. Freud moved away from inducing trance states in his patients via hypnotic suggestion. Instead, he used 'free association.' That is, the patient is told to say everything that comes to mind without censoring, selective editing, or suppression. Freud followed an assumption based on his belief in psychic determinism (that there are cause-effect relations in the mind and that they are connecting all the patient's associations). However, Freud noticed that certain people couldn't be hypnotized. These people appeared to have strong feelings about the doctor that seemed to block the hypnotic process. Freud later turned these observations into processes called resistance (blocking) and transference (feelings about the doctor).

Each of Freud's case histories was written with a specific focus (and 'formulation'); here are a few:

- The *Dora* Case (Freud 1905) was written to show how dreams are used in psychoanalysis.

DOI: 10.4324/9781003375944-2

- *The Rat Man* (Freud 1909) was written to demonstrate the structure of obsessional neurosis.
- *The Wolfman* (Freud 1918) was written as a political commentary. Freud wrote it as his counterargument to Jung's theories. Freud was trying to show exactly how the reconstruction of the patient's infantile sexuality confirms Freud's hypothesis of psychosexual development.

Some suggest that Freud was filled with biases and that he was motivated to find the things that he found. While this might be so, there are now 120 years of amassed clinical and research data, both in psychology and in neuroscience, to suggest that many of Freud's clinical observations are at least partly true.

In the formulation of his cases, Freud also introduced a very important clinical technique: talk therapy. This psychoanalytic technique is comprised of the following:

- Free association
- Detailed inquiry
- Reconstruction
- Interpretation—that is, the process where the therapist correlates the patient's reconstructions to his or her symptoms

That said, with all the brilliance that Freud displayed in these case histories, Fine (1987) suggests that there are several problems with them:

- Many of the patients in *Studies on Hysteria* we would now diagnose as suffering from what Freud called the narcissistic neurosis. Dora, Wolfman, and Rat Man would probably now be diagnosed as borderline personality disorder or mixed neurotic with borderline features.

- A major omission in Freud's case histories is that there is no discussion/analysis of the patient's defenses, that is, the patient's overall character structure. This describes an understanding of a patient's particular defenses, and how they work to protect this person from pain and suffering while ironically causing the person even more pain and suffering. This defensive structure is the person's character as it developed in childhood via identification with the person's early objects. At this point in Freud's work, he was only interested in working with the patient's symptoms, not with the total personality.

As we now know, when talking about a series of defenses the person uses, we're talking about this person's character/personality.

To summarize, what Freud did in his case histories was given as follows:

- He classified the clinical material.
- He correlated the symptoms with infantile sexuality.

- He called this process 'reconstruction.'
- He created the therapeutic techniques of psychoanalysis as a talk therapy.

Freud believed that the processes described in *Hysteria* were the same as what occurs in obsessional neurosis and phobia. However, in the obsessional neurosis—as seen in *The Rat Man* (1909), there is a regression to the anal-sadistic stage of infantile sexuality, and the person struggles with both sexual impulses and sadistic hatred. Following this regression, there is the same failure of repression, breakthrough of repressed impulses, and formation of symptoms. In *The Wolfman* (1918), Freud attempts to show how the process of reconstruction of infantile sexuality confirms Freud's hypothesis of psychosexual development. Freud presented neurosis as an extension of a normal psychical process. Yet, if neurosis is the result of a universal process (i.e., if all human beings employ a certain amount of repression), is everyone neurotic? To understand Freud's answer to this question, we note that Freud was ambivalent about psychology. While Freud made many brilliant psychological observations in his career, he hoped that science would discover a biological underpinning to neurosis. One consequence of this is that whenever Freud couldn't explain a psychological phenomenon psychologically, he'd fall back on a biological explanation. Thus, to the question: Why does one person 'become neurotic,' while another doesn't? Freud answers that neurotics are inherently (biologically) more easily frustrated/more easily gratified at the bodily zones. Because of this inherited predisposition, neurotics are more likely to have strong fixations, more likely to have more frequent and pervasive failures of repression, and therefore more likely to have more frequent neurosis.

While Freud had begun looking at the unconscious threads in his and in Breuer's patient's communications, (cf Breuer and Freud, 1896) the detailed and explicit act of describing how one traces the patient's current issues to the person's childhood conflicts came much later in Freud's work.[2,3]

As we talk throughout this book about case material and particularly about case formulation, as I say to my doctoral and postdoctoral students, I want to mention my belief that every mental health clinician should have at least *some* experiences with hospital work. Although this kind of setting can be emotionally challenging, if your goal is clinic work and/or office practice, and you're not planning to work with seriously disturbed patients, then it's particularly important to have hospital experience and be able to have firsthand knowledge about very disturbed patients who aren't currently functioning. Having experience working with disturbed people is a good way to know how to access those people that need more management and monitoring than office practice allows, versus those who can do well with psychodynamic talk therapy and/or talk therapy and medication. Moreover, as we will see throughout this book, without experience with people who have *too much accessibility* to unconscious processes, it is harder to separate reasonably higher functioning, but perhaps odd people, from those functioning poorly with lower level (psychotic) defenses.

Here is an example:

> I once worked with a young man, a practicing attorney. In the middle of the first interview, during my questioning, this man began to act very oddly. I knew from hospital experiences that he was not psychotic, in the formal sense of blunted affect and thought disorder, but he was certainly *acting crazy.* I also knew I could work with him, but if I hadn't had hospital experience, I don't know that I would have known this. He certainly did odd things. Yet, because of what I had previously learned in terms of affect blunting and/or loss of control over affect, as well as relatedness versus psychotic withdrawal, I had a high degree of confidence that we could work together with what he was presenting.

The episode of what I will now call 'oddness' (actually, an enactment) occurred when he was describing his childhood. He'd said that his parents were always yelling and critical, but when I inquired about this, he said, "Like this," and then, he started yelling at the top of his voice and making barely recognizable howling sounds like a ferocious creature.

I want to be clear: what he did was very odd. I'm not suggesting otherwise. It was odd enough for me to go back into my mental files about hospitalized patients, to say to myself:

> no blunted affect, makes eye contact, tolerated it when I moved my chair just a bit closer to him, had a coherent description of his history, had until this point in the intake interview manifested the ability to test reality.

He had also, by the way, graduated from an excellent college and law school, but that data might lead one to only draw conclusions about his *prior* level of functioning: I had to plan about how he was acting at present. After a few seconds of this yelling, he sat back in his chair and reassured me that, while he had been making weird sounds:

> I don't usually act like this.

Thus, I observed that he had critical ego functions in that he was able to describe what he had done. (In regard to this yelling and making weird sounds, I suggested to him that this behavior made him seem unattractive and a bit frightening. I also suggested that perhaps his acting unpredictable and irrational had been a tactic that he developed in childhood to protect himself from being killed by his toxic family. While he neither confirmed nor denied my remark, he then went on to describe how none of his three siblings had fared as well as he had in their own lives. That felt like a preconscious confirmation of what I'd just said, and later work with this man was also confirmatory of these preliminary thoughts about him.)

Additionally, I remember presenting this case and my understanding of it to one of my doctoral classes, where one student said the following about my very quick interpretation of this man's odd behavior:

… Your comments sounded poetically beautiful, but how do you know whether they had anything to do with this patient?[4]

Here was my reply at the time:

I didn't have great confidence that my comments were accurate/near accurate/ or off the mark. This is one of the important things that we will be talking about throughout this book; that even in Freud's case histories - where he introduces the technique of reconstruction (that is, taking the person's current symptoms, character traits and defenses - and reconstructing what kind of history the person might have had based on their current adjustment and symptomatology and behavior in the session) we can never be sure that our *magical* guesses are correct until we accrue more data that confirms or disconfirms our provisional understanding.

At the time of this class, I also added that my comments might not be something that these students wanted to hear, because new clinicians desire certainty. I will be returning to this point, and its profound implications, throughout this book.

That said, this is the essence of what you be learning from me—how to make (increasingly) *educated guesses* about the dynamics and historical origin of a person's current suffering.

All humans have a psychology that is largely based upon their psychological development, such questions as: At what age was this person exposed to trauma? What were they like *pre-morbid* (before the trauma)? How much, if at all, did the person collude in the trauma? (This is a very delicate question that can make it seem like we are *blaming the victim*, when in fact, no matter how much a person may have colluded with their traumatizer, it is always the fault of the traumatizer rather than the person who was traumatized.) What sources of support were available to the traumatized person, and was the person able to use these resources? And, if they were not able to use these resources, then why weren't they able to? Just as we will see with the issue of the presenting problem, everything that we hypothesize in every clinical session with a patient is true and may not be quite true at the same time.

Here is another example.

I once performed an intake interview with a disbarred attorney who was now planning a scheme to embezzle money in stock transactions. This is what I reconstructed, based on his arrogant, contemptuous, and demeaning behavior toward me.

This man had had a very difficult childhood. His mother had been very nasty to him; his father was never around, and, while this man never said so directly, he made it clear that in his mind he believed he had the right to swindle money. I listened for the entire session without commenting (this is unusual for me). Then, I said there would be no charge for the session because I didn't think I had much of value to add to what he already believed.

He said: "You don't have any advice for me?"

I now said the following:

> I told him that I didn't feel that I could work with him because it seemed that he was very much identified with a mother who was a 'nasty bitch' as a mother, and it seemed as if his father had been no protection for him, and that during our session, he had acted just like his mother: that he had been a nasty bitch to me. But, worse than that, it seemed as if he was on his way to becoming a 'nasty bitch' to himself. That, if one's wishes always came true like they do in fairy tales, he could become rich with his plan, but I doubted it. And I thought that one way he was a 'nasty bitch' to himself was that he was going to wind up in prison.

He listened intently and then, as if he hadn't taken in a word I said, he repeated: "But you still haven't given me any advice."

I said: "Well, I don't want to be harsh to you, so I have been holding myself back to not repeat your childhood relationships, to not be a nasty bitch to you. But, if you want advice, then here it is: You should take martial arts lessons."
He said: "What's so good about martial arts?"
I said: "Because I think that you're going to wind up in prison. You can use martial arts to defend yourself."

By using this example, I want to demonstrate the following, and prepare all of you for what's ahead: the clinician's job, as I understand it, is to use all data, including reconstruction, to make meaning in the therapy. Equally important to what the person has told you about their history is how they are treating you, the therapist. This man was treating me as if he was embezzling me. I let this happen (no charge for the session) because, underneath this, he was filled (in a kind of identification with his mother) with a compensatory grandiosity, omnipotence, and disdain for others. By telling him that he was unworkable with talk therapy, I was attempting to create meaning with a person who was intent on making the session meaningless (because for him, any meaning that occurred would have made him feel awful about his life). Of course, there was a part of me that hoped against hope that he could be shocked into being interested in what I had to say and that he would want to actually receive some of the wisdom I believed I could offer him. In fact, in this regard, I did do a bit of therapy with him, even during the very brief time that we met, and even though I'd told him I wasn't going to. That is, I made a few trial interpretations ("nasty bitch to yourself") that could have brought meaning into the session, but he refused it. As a follow-up, I was saddened to hear, about a year later, that this man had been arrested, charged, convicted of fraud, and sentenced to a long-term imprisonment.

From Freud to Wilhelm Reich

Wilhelm Reich—Character Analysis (1946)

Wilhelm Reich published his only major psychoanalytic work, the groundbreaking book, *Charakteranalyse* in 1933; it was revised and published in English in 1946 and 1949 as *Character Analysis*. This book sought to move psychoanalysis toward what Reich called a reconfiguration of character structure.

For Reich, character structure is the result of social processes, in particular a reflection of the Oedipal anxieties that are the *result* of conflicts within each nuclear family.

Reich proposed that a kind of *muscular armor* develops within each person's body and serves as a defense that contains within it the history of the persons' childhood traumas. For example, Reich suggests that Freud's jaw cancer was caused by his muscular armor, rather than by his cigar smoking: Freud's Judaism meant he was 'biting down' impulses, rather than expressing his hatred because he faced a virulent and continual anti-Semitism. To Reich, dissolving the armor would bring back memories of Freud's childhood repression that had caused the blockage in the first place.[5]

Reich's new technical approach to psychoanalytic treatment caused a shift from the exclusive study of unconscious material obtained through free association, to a focus on the patient's *character*, that is, a focus on his/her characteristic behavior used to defend against the psychoanalyst's insight and against the unconscious material. This shift in emphasis helped to make formerly inaccessible patients now analyzable and put an end to long, depressing, psychoanalyses of many years' duration *with a wealth of material but no mobilizing of the patient's feelings.* Reich suggested that these feelings are always bound up within the patient's *character armor*. Thus, with this new approach, Reich suggested that there was no longer a need for 'the therapeutic alibi':

...The patient just doesn't want to get well...
...He/she (the patient) is using the illness as a punishment....

Reich elaborated on Freud's insight that every neurotic disorder is a conflict between repressed instinctual demands and the repressing forces of the ego. However, he added that making conscious what had been unconscious needs to occur indirectly, by eliminating the patient's resistance; this is the key to the resolution of the neurosis. The patient must first find out *that* he/she defends himself/herself, and then, *by what means* that he/she defends himself/herself, and only then, the patient can find *against what he/she is defending.*

Thus, the psychotherapist does not interpret the patient's material as it emerges via free association. Reich believes that Freud was not correct; *patients are unable to follow the basic rule of free association!* Instead, it is essential to comprehend and work with the patient's transference resistances. What the psychoanalyst needs to understand and work with is more about whether or not the patient is deceiving you; and/or whether or not he/she has a secret attitude of derision toward you; and/or whether or not he/she is blocked and blunted in affect.

From Reich, we see an emphasis not only on what patient *does and says* but also on what *is not done and not said.* This is what Reich calls latent resistances. In essence, what Reich is saying is that Freud's idea of the basic rule was fine; however, it's just that no one can easily follow it! As an example of what Reich is talking about, I remind you of the case presented above: the disbarred attorney/embezzler. Here my technique centered on pointing out the patient's uncooperativeness that was being hidden under the rubble of his contempt and disdain for me and for the process of therapy—and underneath that, a contempt for himself.

Latent Negative Resistance: It's easier to see negative transference, and what appears like positive transference, at the beginning of therapy, but all of this can be a narcissistic transference reaction that is not, in fact, a positive transference. That is, the patient acts cooperatively because he/she thinks you love them (the therapist is acting interested and supportive). However, when the patient realizes that you don't love them but that you are being kind because this is your *job*, the transference becomes negative. Or there is another possibility as with my embezzler patient—the negative resistance is barely hidden. Or it is more carefully hidden—but negative.

Reich describes several types of hidden (latent) negative resistances:

- Over obedient, friendly, too trusting, 'overly good' passive character
- Conventional and correct compulsive, that is, a person that converts hatred into politeness
- Affect lame, that is, a person who is blocking their aggressivity
- Inward smile, that is, a 'phony'—what has been called an 'as if personality' (Deutsch 1942) which means a person who seems to have no substance/identity, but who—underneath the falseness—is both narcissistic and contemptuous

In sum, Reich's major technical innovation is that he suggests that the therapist must shift from an emphasis on *content* to an emphasis on the *latent negative resistances.* In other words, the clinician works with the resistance and then the material follows—*instead of the reverse.*

Here Is an Example of How Psychodynamic Therapy Technique Is Modified by Reich's Approach

A patient (young man) loved his mother and idealized her, and he felt helpless and impotent in the presence of his competent by undermining, shaming, and arrogant father.

In the therapy, the patient would continually say to the therapist:

I just can't think of anything to say…

The therapist began to believe that the patient was creating a situation where both the patient and the therapist would feel impotent—just as the patient had felt as a child (this is an *enactment*), but now the therapist (as a substitute for the father of the patient's childhood) would feel impotent as well.

The therapist began to focus his questions on the patient's fantasies about this therapist's failings: he asked the patient to imagine what kind of therapist is unable to help a man like the patient, when that man is in such distress.

The patient now expressed rage at the therapist for:

…Making this all about you…

After this outburst, the patient began to share memories of childhood wishes that his father had been weak, impotent, and a failure and that the father would have had a *taste* of what he was doing to his son.

Reich's approach, as presented in this vignette, helped to lead to many innovations in psychoanalytic technique. In fact, Otto Kernberg[6] has cited Reich's contribution of the analysis of character to Kernberg's own technical approach in the psychotherapy of patients suffering from 'borderline personality disorder.'

From Wilhelm Reich to Theodore Reik

Theodore Reik (1948, 1959)[6]

I will now devote a significant amount of time to the work of Theodore Reik. I do this for three reasons: first, I was fortunate to have had a personal experience with Dr. Reik; he had mentored my aunt, in the early 1950s/1960s (my mother's sister Mildred Newman). Mildred Newman became Dr. Reik's protégé, and most importantly, I also learned a lot about him and his work, starting from the time that I was a very young boy. Also, and for a less prosaic reason, Reik's work is very relevant to the work of many modern psychoanalytic approaches, and yet, he is almost unknown to mainstream psychoanalysis (see Arnold 2006).[3] Thus, there are many similarities with Reik's work and later developments in psychodynamic psychotherapy, such as Relational Psychoanalysis, as well as with several non-psychodynamic models, such as the works of both Carl Rogers (1961) and Jay

Haley (1963, 1973). Finally, Reik's work on *confession* is particularly relevant to how I understand the processes that occur in case formulation and to the processes that occur in a *case presentation*.

Theodore Reik earned his Ph.D. degree in psychology from the University of Vienna (where Freud had studied medicine) in 1912. Reik's dissertation was only the second psychoanalytic dissertation written, coming one year after one penned by Dr. Otto Rank. After receiving his doctorate, Reik devoted several years to studying with Freud. Freud financially supported Reik and his family during this time, while Reik was himself psychoanalyzed by another of Freud's early students, Dr. Karl Abraham. Reik's first major book was *The Compulsion to Confess* (1925), in which he argued that neurotic symptoms such as blushing and stuttering could be seen as unconscious confessions that express the patient's repressed impulses while, at the same time, punishing the patient for communicating these impulses. Reik further explored this theme in *The Unknown Murderer* (1932), in which he examined the process of psychologically profiling unknown criminals. Reik argued that because of unconscious guilt, criminals often leave clues that can lead to their identification and arrest. That said, Reik's most important book, *Listening with the Third Ear* (Reik 1948), describes how psychoanalysts intuitively use their own unconscious minds to decipher the unconscious of their patients. As one will soon surmise, this is key to my understanding of the processes that occur in case presentations.

Kyle Arnold (2006),[6] in a very thoughtful and comprehensive paper about Reik's work, suggests that Reik expressed one fundamental belief: *human beings have a basic need to express 'ourselves to others.'* Thus, the child's expressions develop as compromises between the urge to express and the internalized responses of his/her caregivers to expressions, and these internalized responses are continually consolidated into the child's superego. When/if others repeatedly reject the child's expressions, then the child comes to reject his/her own expressions through repression. Repressed expressions return as composites of the need to express and internalized prohibitions against expression. These composites emerge as *unconscious confessions* in which the patient both communicates repressed material and punishes himself/herself for doing so. Reik proposes that neurotic symptoms comprise such unconscious confessions. In this regard, as I have presented above, Reik cites a famous passage of "A Fragment of an Analysis of a Case of Hysteria" (The Dora Case) where Freud writes that:

> He that has eyes to see and ears to hear may convince himself that no mortal can keep a secret. If his lips are silent, he chatters with his fingertips; betrayal oozes out of him at every pore.
>
> (1905/1953, pp. 77–78)

Arnold (2006) suggests that Freud and Reik are both alluding to the inability of mortals to keep their unconscious secrets from others, a thesis that supports the scientific and clinical edifice of psychoanalysis (Reik 1925/1959b, p. 187).

Psychoanalysis works because, in the long run, mortals cannot hide, at least not from their psychoanalysts. A somewhat less obvious implication of the passage, however, is that we all carry a deep-seated urge to express our hidden wishes and fantasies to others. From this perspective, symptoms and the so-called Freudian slips are aimed at exposure, 'betrayal' of one's secrets and confessions. In other words, Reik suggests, mortals are unable to keep secrets because deep down, we do not want to.

Arnold (2006) offers that Freud's own work never fully realizes this notion. To be sure, Freud often asserts that unconscious wishes strive for discharge. In this sense, wishes push for expression, for if they are to be discharged, they must emerge in some form. Yet, from Freud's perspective, the expression of wishes to others is more of a mere secondary effect of discharge (rather than a goal in and of itself). To Reik, we all possess a deeply rooted need to express ourselves to others. This need inevitably comes into conflict with the prohibitions of the external world as well as the prohibitions of the superego. Consequently, we repress and suppress much of ourselves. However, the need to express remains operative in the unconscious, driving us to unwittingly convey our most unacceptable wishes despite our inhibitions. Because such expressions are experienced as forbidden, we can only express our unconscious secrets while also punishing ourselves for doing so. Thus, the expression of dynamically unconscious material takes the form of a composite of self-expression and self-punishment. Reik calls that composite *confession* and proposes that it comprises the basic structure of neurotic symptoms (1925/1959b, p. 348).

Here Is an Example of the Processes That Reik Describes

Some years ago, a colleague told me about a new case of his; he had just begun to treat a surgeon who had been caught shoplifting and had been arrested and was now, as a condition of his release, under court remand to be treated by this clinician. It seems that this doctor needed a letter to the courts to attest that he was in psychological treatment and to both attest to his good character and offer that this offense was just a one-time error in judgment. My somewhat bewildered clinician/friend sought out my advice because he said that he thought that I could be helpful in *making meaning* out of an act that seemed, on its face, *so senseless*. This therapist wondered what I thought about this, particularly given that the man didn't need money and that what this patient had stolen amounted to trinkets of almost no value. I made some suggestions to my colleague, and a few days later, my colleague/ friend called to thank me and report, with some surprise, that I seemed to understand all of this. In fact, he had had the following conversation with his patient:

My colleague to his patient:

> "I wanted to ask you, did you recently get a promotion or other professional honor before your arrest for shoplifting…?"

Patient:

> "...Did my lawyer tell you about that...I was just made Chief of XX (specialty) at my hospital...wait he (the lawyer) couldn't have told you...I never told him that...how did you know this?"

This colleague then explained that he 'didn't know it' but that he had surmised that something *good* had happened to this man and that, because of the patient's childhood history, the patient would have needed to punish himself if he was feeling too much pride and/or success. That is, given the patient's history and psychodynamics, after a success, this patient might be filled with feelings of guilt as well as filled with a powerful need to express *both the guilt* and *the need to be punished for it*. What better way to express that he felt both 'bad' and 'guilty' than to be caught *in the act of being* bad and guilty about *something?* These comments led the patient to talk about issues of guilt as well as the issue of *shame* as important dynamics in the patient's childhood family. And, further, *that as a child he had sometimes committed silly acts of what he called 'badness'* whenever he had been feeling 'too good' about himself.

Following Reik's reasoning, it appears that, along with the urge to discharge tension and achieve pleasure, human beings are endowed with what Reik calls "an independent emotional tendency" to express ourselves to others (1925/1959b, p. 193). To be sure, Reik claims that the infant's earliest "expressions of drives"—such as "screaming, crying, and thrashing about" (p. 193)—originally serve only the function of "motor discharge" (p. 193). Nevertheless, such expressions rapidly become "the representation and communication of our needs to the external world as a kind of invitation to accomplish gratification" (p. 197). Although the desire for drive gratification and the urge for expression serve somewhat different functions (p. 193), these functions are interconnected. We cannot get what we want without expressing it to others, and without any urges to communicate, we would have nothing substantive to express. "We want to talk of the things which constitute our wishing and longing," Reik (p. 312) writes, for "if we cannot talk about these, what sense does talking make?" For Reik, then, motivation has both one-person (drive gratification) and two-person (object relations) dimensions.

Confession

Reik claims that repression strengthens the need to express. Thus, the more expressions are muted, the less the need to express will be met and the more urgent it will become (pp. 185, 197). *Secret Knowledge*, as Reik (1932, p. 49) puts it, "clamors to be revealed." However, because the repressed need to express remains active despite the superego's prohibition against communication, it is modified by guilt and the need for punishment. Reik claims that repression, once again, is motivated by social anxiety internalized as guilt. Guilt inhibits free expression (Reik 1925, pp. 223–224). Paradoxically, though, guilt also motivates the compulsion to confess (pp. 201, 204, 309). According to Reik (following Freud), unconscious guilt carries with it a need for punishment (pp. 292–293). The need to relieve guilt by provoking punishment adds to the confession's compulsive quality, for the more guilt one feels about what one wants to express, the more one will be compelled to convey it to others so that they will get *the punishment they deserve.* This seems to have been very clear in my colleague's case of the physician (presented above). And I will later develop this notion further to suggest that these same processes Reik describes in symptom formation and in many other types of communication are also relevant to the *pressures* felt by the Presenter in the clinical presentation.

Types of Confession

Arnold emphasizes that for Reik, guilt not only contributes to the confession's compulsive quality but may also influence the form taken by the confession. Reik describes three major varieties of confession that correspond to varying degrees of guilt. He argues that the more guilt the patient is attempting to contain, the more pathological the form that the confessions will take. Increased guilt corresponds both to increased repression and increased need for punishment, and therefore, the comparatively guilty patient will make confessions that are more distorted, compulsive, and self-destructive than those of a patient whose guilt is less profound. In this regard, the surgeon who was arrested for shoplifting would be a dramatic example of the enactment of a *self-destructive guilty confession via an enactment.*

Conscious Verbal Confession

If guilt is not very strong and it is being consciously suppressed rather than unconsciously repressed, a confession can be made verbally and consciously. *Conscious verbal confession* is the kind of confession with which we are most familiar.

Unconscious Verbal Confession and Enacted Confession

When unconscious guilt reaches a certain threshold, Reik proposes, forbidden impulses are exhibited in behavior rather than expressed verbally. As Reik (1925/1959b, p. 207) puts it, "the impulse to replace reproduction in narration by acting-out appears especially when the events to be reproduced are under the pressure of a particularly strong feeling of guilt." Nonverbal confessions express "forbidden tendencies" by "demonstrating" them (Reik 1957, p. 205). The structure of unconscious confession outlined above still holds—an enacted confession, like an unconscious verbal confession, expresses and disguises repressed wishes while punishing the patient for that expression—*but the patient shows what he or she is guilty about rather than telling others about it.*

BTW, I believe, and we will soon see, that it is not only the patient that enacts a guilty confession. Much of what we will be witnessing in this book are examples of our therapist/Presenters making *enacted guilty confessions* via the expression of gratuitous remarks that serve as clues to both the patient's and the therapist's conflictual thoughts/feelings and guilt. Reik offers two reasons why this occurs. For one thing, because guilt motivates repression, when guilt is particularly strong, repression will be especially powerful. Furthermore, as consciousness is closely connected to language, the more a guilt-ridden expression is driven into the unconscious, the less likely it will be to emerge verbally. To be communicated, deeply repressed impulses might only appear nonverbally. Second, the stronger the patient's (or therapist's) guilt, the greater the need for punishment will be. Under the pressure of an intensified need for punishment, the patient (or, I suggest, the therapist/Presenter) may be compelled to behave in a self-sabotaging way, expecting that doing so will maximize the punishment that he or she will receive. Thus, "precisely as the need for punishment increases the acting-out appears especially lively" (p. 209). In all these acts, the patient is simultaneously expressing forbidden tendencies while also punishing himself or herself for that expression!

In other words, for Reik, repression is a repetition of childhood ruptures in communication. Repressed expressions return as composites of the urge to express and internalized prohibitions against expression. The internalized social anxieties linked to the superego both inhibit free expression and produce a need for punishment. Neurotic symptoms are *confessions* that combine unconscious expression with self-punishment (Arnold 2006).

I will now summarize and apply Reik's ideas both to more recent work in psychoanalysis and to my own current work.

Recent Work in Psychoanalysis and Psychotherapy

Aspects of Reik's work can be seen in the later writings of both Carl Rogers (1961) and Heinz Kohut (2009). Rogers (1961) was a humanistic psychotherapist and not a psychoanalyst, and one can see in his work what he called: *childhood conditions of worth*. That is, as children we quickly learn to hide those thoughts and feelings that we view to be unacceptable to our parents. In the development of the self-concept, Rogers saw conditional and unconditional positive regard as key. Those raised in an environment of unconditional positive regard can fully actualize themselves. Those raised in an environment of *conditional positive regard* feel worthy only if they match the conditions (what Rogers describes as *conditions of worth*) that had been laid down for them by others. In other words, these children, and later these same adults, hide their true feelings from expression—first to others and later even to themselves.

In the work of Kohut (2009), we see that the lack of parental empathy leads the developing child to a regression, that is, into a narcissistic retreat from contact with others. Kohut demonstrated his interest in how we develop our "sense of self" using narcissism as a model. If a person is narcissistic, he/she will allow themselves to suppress feelings of low self-esteem. By withholding the expression of the unacceptable parts of the self and only talking highly of *the acceptable self*, the person can maintain his/her sense of worthiness (and *hide any sense of worthlessness*).

In sum, Reik's observations suggest that we humans have a deep need to communicate our deepest parts to others. Further, his observations lend support to my own theory of preconscious communication. This understanding has led to me a detailed study of the processes involved in *confession*, and most importantly, it has influenced my own understanding of the value of what I have previously labeled: a Presenter's *gratuitous remarks* (seemingly random remarks that occur during a clinical presentation that are in fact rich with preconscious/conflictual meaning). In other words, Reik's ideas help to explain what we will see in the many ways that clinician/Presenters seem to be compelled to tell all of what they have experienced with their patient—their conscious experiences as well as their preconscious ones. That is, my focus during a presentation of clinical material has often been one that, at first blush, might appear to be seemingly irrelevant and superfluous. Just as one might watch closely for the patient's slips of the tongue and errors of omission and commission in a psychoanalytic psychotherapy session, I view all seemingly 'off-the-cuff comments' (as well as other so-called random comments, mistakes, and slips of the tongue) that are made by the Presenter during the clinical presentation as *the* road to travel in my quest to arrive at the very *heart and soul of every clinical enterprise.*

As we will see throughout this book, I believe that the conflict between the wish/need to express and the wish/need to hide occurs for a variety of reasons in a patient during every clinical encounter. That said, I also believe that there *is a similar process that can also be seen in the 'compromises' that occur inside of the presenting clinician during his/her clinical presentation.* In other words, what I am suggesting is that a sense of shame/guilt and fear in the Presenter can lead to conflicts that result in ambivalence and that this ambivalence can be *seen and understood* in the translation of latent material in the clinician's presentation. And, further, it is this ambivalence that is sometimes (I would even suggest *typically*) enacted in many, if not all, clinical presentations.

A Question Might Now Come to Mind

Given what I have presented to you so far, it might be reasonable for each of you to ask, then, what is the reason(s) that I believe that a Presenter might feel ambivalent (shameful/guilty) about the very act of presentation, and even more curious, why might a Presenter feel unconscious guilt/shame and fear about knowing what they know and how they know it? Is this the guilt/shame and fear that is related to feelings about the Patient/about the Consultant/about the Current Supervisor/about all the above? It is, in fact, often about all of this! However, I contend that there is also another (powerful and not conscious) reason that a Presenter might be ambivalent about presenting clinical material: I believe that the very act of presenting clinical material to a group of clinicians, particularly when one is a student, can encourage one to feel like an *expert*.

That is, I contend that in each clinician, there lies a combination of fear, shame, and guilt connected to what a clinical presentation means: mixed feelings about knowing what you know and knowing that you can decipher *what it is that you don't yet know.* Further, I contend that all of this has to do with mixed feelings about the *danger* of being seen as omnipotent! If I am correct about this, it would make even more sense that when a bit of clinical information is not quite clear—that is, when it is *preconscious*—a clinician might feel that it is presumptuous of him/her to attempt to read into this information any vague/poorly formed notions about the dynamics of a patient for fear that he/she will appear to be acting like an *omnipotent magician.*

After so many years of doing just this, that is, doing exactly what I have just described, and doing it well, that is, being accurate for a good deal of the time, I no longer have such constraints.

To continue, if one follows my logic further, perhaps therefore it is easier to see 'me,' the Consultant, as an omnipotent magician *rather than to see this whole endeavor as both a teachable and learnable way to become clinically powerful.* After all, this is an endeavor that is centered on unraveling the mysteries of the mind. And arrogance is not an attractive trait, and further, it is even harder to be arrogant when one is presenting ideas about vague/unstructured/ephemeral processes. It is perhaps better to project *omnipotence and magic* into *another.*

To summarize, Reik's ideas have also influenced me to develop a technique of clinical consultation that often results in the Presenter *wanting to believe* that what I do is *magical.* Further, I contend that the belief that I am *magical* is emotionally easier for many Presenters than to believe that the techniques I perform are both teachable and learnable; that is, it is easier to believe that I can perform *magic* than to believe that any clinician can learn the same *magic* and therefore can learn to be, in this poetic sense, *omnipotent.* I will later demonstrate that when we want to make meaning out of each clinical case, we can and should use every bit of data that emerges. In this regard, the group setting is the best place to see this via the interchanges that, as we will soon see, take place among the members.

Finally, as Arnold (2006) points out, there are similarities between the ideas of Theodore Reik and the recent ideas of *Relational Psychoanalysis.* I would also suggest that Reik's ideas also have some similarities with the later understanding of several non-psychoanalytic clinicians, who focused their ideas on the communication properties of language in psychotherapy. Included here are the works of Carl Rogers (1961) (see above), Milton Erickson, (c f Haley 1963), and Jay Haley (1973) (see below).

From Theodore Reik to D.W. Winnicott (1964) and W.R. Bion (1962, 1976)

Winnicott's (1964) concept of the therapist co-creating and holding open a bridge between internal and external reality, and thus offering a transitional space, resulted from his pediatric work with children and their mothers. This work led to the development of the influential concept that he called the 'holding environment.' Winnicott claimed that the foundations of health are laid down by the ordinary mother in her ordinary loving care of her own baby and that central to this care was the mother's attentive holding of her child.

Winnicott considered that the "mother's technique of holding, of bathing, of feeding, everything she did for the baby, added up to the child's first idea of the mother," as well as fostering the ability to experience the body as the place where one securely lives. Extrapolating the concept of holding from mother to the family and to the outside world, Winnicott saw as key to healthy development, "the continuation of reliable holding in terms of the ever-widening circle of family and school and social life".

Winnicott was influential in viewing the work of the psychotherapist as offering a substitute holding environment based on the mother/infant bond. Winnicott wrote:

> A correct and well-timed interpretation in an analytic treatment gives a sense of being held physically that is more real...than if a real holding or nursing had taken place. Understanding goes deeper.

Further, Winnicott's theoretical writings emphasized empathy, imagination, and the highly particular transactions that constitute love between two people. This concept parallels the work on rupture and repair in psychoanalytic therapy (Castonguay & Muran 2016) and is at the heart of my understanding of how/why clinicians present their data to their supervisors and consultants. In other words, at the heart of the way student/Presenters present their cases is:

> the hidden fact that the Presenter conveys more than they are consciously aware that they are conveying, thereby creating the false narrative that the Consultant/ supervisor is performing a kind of clinical magic, just as the mother 'performs magic' by holding her baby.

Bion's (1962) presented a valuable concept of the mother or therapist, who in his/ her reverie and via his/her alpha functioning is transmitting to the acutely distressed baby (or as therapist they are conveying to their patient) the seeds of the capacity to think rather than to evacuate the thoughts. This growing capacity is, in some ways, like Winnicott's 'holding,' although Winnicott's concept seems to involve a less active and perhaps less intrusive process on the part of the mother, one that is very protective of the child's fragile ego.

Bion's idea of maternal 'reverie' as the capacity to sense (and make sense of) what is going on inside the infant has been an important element in my own current understanding of the patient/therapist conscious and preconscious transactions. Reverie is an act of faith in the unconscious process... essential to alpha-function. It is considered the equivalent of Winnicott's maternal preoccupation.

In therapy, the clinician's use of 'reverie' is an important tool in his/her response to the patient's material: It is this capacity for *playing with a patient's images* that Bion encouraged (Symington & Symington 1996), *and it is what I look for in the gratuitous remarks/slips of the tongue/other data in the interaction between myself (the Consultant) and the clinician* (the Presenter). In this regard, as with my life experience with Theodore Reik, I had the 'once-in-a-lifetime' opportunity to see the processes that Bion wrote about in action, that is, in my supervision with him in 1976! To have witnessed the power of 'reverie' and his skill in being able to decode the preconscious transactions in the most complicated of clinical situations was a 'life-changing' event for me, and it is another influence that has led me down the current path that I am now presenting in this book.

In sum, I suggest that the very process of creating a *holding environment where the clinician can find a safe space for reverie* also makes that same clinician vulnerable to the patient's projections/projective identifications and enactments, all of which are typically not accessible to the clinician's conscious awareness. Yet, at the same time, this preconscious experience also creates a pressure for its conscious expression (Reik 1948).

When this same clinician becomes a Presenter, particularly when their Consultant is skilled at creating an atmosphere wherein the Presenter feels both held and allowed to be *in reverie*, the result is often a heightened pull *to express and confess*. In fact, we have already seen bits of this above, and we will soon be seeing a good deal more below in even greater detail. Further, as part of the creation of a 'holding place for reverie,' a skilled Consultant can often become quite attuned to these processes by continually being alert to them. In a similar fashion to the skill building that occurs in the making of an experienced clinician, a skilled Consultant/ Supervisor will over time develop a 'well-stocked mind' (Shulman 1982) that makes the creation of a space for holding/reverie, and the facile making and testing of clinical hypotheses, a relatively straightforward endeavor.

In this regard, *Psychoanalytic Epistemology* asks questions such as "How do you know?" "What does it mean to say that you know something?"[7] What makes you *believe* that the rightness of what you know is justified?" and "How do you know what you know"? In this regard, I want to remind the reader that what I always suggest is a *provisional hypothesis* about any clinical endeavor. That said, the above questions are important for psychoanalysis. Freud avoided addressing such questions of interpretation because they stirred up a conflict for him regarding his positivist scientific ideals. However, as Shulman suggests, writers in psychoanalysis have not successfully incorporated a shift in the epistemology of psychoanalytic science into their approaches to an in-depth psychological understanding. Scientific knowledge in many fields where interpretation plays an important role is not dependent on controlled studies, but rather upon the care with which multiple and redundant checks are applied as work proceeds. The clinical psychoanalyst recognizes how this error-checking process is so much a part of their daily work.[8]

Do experienced psychoanalysts have a special kind of expertise? Studies of expertise in many fields have shown that the most important difference between experts and individuals who are less successful in their fields is *their extensive detailed knowledge*, which permits them to focus on problem solution rather than following a set method. Problem-solving strategies employed by such experts tend to be carried out with considerable flexibility. The experts don't use cognitive methods identifiably different from those used by others; rather, they demonstrate what Schulman called a 'well-stocked mind.' Yet, it is rare that the exact nature of the expertise can be stated in many fields, as in psychoanalysis or in psychoanalytic supervision/case formulation. The clinical situation, where the psychoanalyst has an extensive and wide exposure to the mind and life of each long-term patient, constitutes a very special form of expertise about each patient that is often generalizable to many patients and that has been both underestimated and not been studied carefully.

From Winnicott and Bion to Billow and Mendelsohn (1987, 1990)

In the late 1980s and into the 1990s, my colleague (Dr. Richard Billow) and I began to explore the complex processes of transference and countertransference that occur early in a therapy, even in the early minutes of an initial interview. In *The Interviewer's Presenting Problems in the Initial Interview* (1990), we suggested that it is not only *the patient* who has presenting problems at a first interview but also in fact the *interviewer* has his or her own 'presenting problems,' as well.

Here's an example of one kind of presenting problem: A young male (or female) *interviewer* is starting a clinical psychotherapy practice, has a doctorate in a mental health specialty, has a couple of years of postdoctoral experience, and has just opened an office; this clinician is feeling excited to start a private clinical practice. Let's say, in this example, it is a male clinician, and he receives a call from a respected senior male colleague, who had been one of this clinician's supervisors several years before. This *senior colleague* says the following:

> I'm working with (supervising) a guy who reminds me of you, at your early training when I worked with you. I'm working with him in supervision. He's delightful, eager to learn, he's smart like you… he's terrific. I want to send him for therapy, he needs a lower fee and I thought that since you are just starting your practice, you might consider this-are you willing?

Well, not only are you willing, but you are also both delighted and thrilled!

However, here's *your* (the new clinician's) presenting problem: This new patient, *highly praised by your former supervisor*, arrives for the first meeting. The first thing he does is growl about the terrible directions that you gave him to the office. (In this way, the navigation apps that are now available have made it much harder to give *directions to one's office*. In the past, one way to assess how well a new patient might *take directions* in therapy was to give extremely clear and accurate directions and wait to see if and how your new patient had *taken your directions*. That is, this seemingly innocuous *direction giving* might have been employed to gather information about the new patient, and in this case, it was.) The new patient now sits down and starts questioning you about your credentials; he seems nasty and quite defensive.

Now, this is *your* (the clinician's) *presenting problem:*

Who is your new patient? Is it the guy that your respected senior supervisor/now colleague called you about, or is it the person that is now seated across from you? Who's your patient? That's this clinician's presenting problem!

This man in front of the clinician seems nothing like the way he was introduced to you over the phone by your supervisor!

Now, one possible *solution* to *your presenting problem* would be to become convinced that your previous supervisor has gone senile and that he is, in fact, now quite out of his mind. Yet, that doesn't really sound right, because the former supervisor was very thoughtful on the phone, and you saw him at a meeting recently and he was making a lot of sense.

Well, then, here's another *solution:* Perhaps you're not yet polished and skilled enough to practice independently, and this new patient (a person beginning in the field and thus probably a clinically sensitive person) saw right through you. And what you experienced and thought you understood about him was, in fact, inaccurate. Yet, that doesn't sound right, either.

So, what is going on here?

What is going on is that you have stumbled upon an important clinical truth: There are two patients in this situation or there might soon be three (in fact, what I am saying is that there is one person, who has different aspects to his/her presentation). The *first patient* is the person that your former supervisor described, and this person acted the way he did with this older, respected colleague. The *second patient* is the person that you saw aggressive, competitive, and contemptuous/devaluing.

With this in mind, here are some common errors that a clinician might make: If one stays focused on what the supervisor told you, and you ignore what has occurred in front of you, I might label this an obsessive-compulsive style, bogged down and blocked by old prior details. If, on the contrary, one drops everything he or she was told and is only concerned with what one sees now, that is, only lives in this current clinical moment; one might suggest that this is a hysterical and/or manic style. Thus, *the interviewer's* presenting problem is that he or she is going to need to find a way to incorporate both what he/she had been told *and* what he/she currently sees before them into a new *real patient.* That new real patient is going to be *some combination of both other patients.*

Why am I bringing this up in relation to this current Case Formulation endeavor? Because either of these styles, obsessive-compulsive or hysterical/manic, will have at least one negative result: *it will inhibit the clinician's curiosity.* Once we lose our curiosity, we limit what it is that we can discover about our patient. It is hard to *make psychological meaning* out of each clinical situation without a curiosity and openness to all aspects of the clinical encounter, and therefore, it will be much harder to understand, and thus help, one's patient.

From this early work with Billow, I soon began to focus (re-focus) on the subtle, and not so-subtle, processes that occur in the preconscious transactions between the therapist and his/her patient (Mendelsohn et al. 1992, 2009). This was the origin of the work that is often now labeled by my students and colleagues as my *clinical magic*.

An Anecdote about Openly Accepting One's Clinical Expertise

After many years of teaching psychoanalytic theory and practice (Mendelsohn 2022) and following only a few class meetings with each new class of beginning doctoral candidates in clinical psychology in my course at Adelphi University—a survey of Freud's theories as seen via a 21st century lens—some version of the following often occurs:

I have typically just made some comment about some clinical matter-making meaning out of something that seemed to make no sense by *decoding preconscious transactions in this or that clinical example.* At this point in my lecture, one member of the class (typically acting as an *unconscious* representative of the rest of the class) will raise his/her hand and ask me the following:

"...Can you read our minds...?"

For many years, I would demur...back off...minimize what I do. However now, I will answer the question in the following truthful way:
Me:

"...*Sure*, I can, but why would I want to?"

Often, at this point, some students gasp.
I now continue:

> "However, if any of you really want me to *read your mind*...BTW, what this means—as you will soon see; if you want me to be looking for the preconscious roots in any of your communications, then this is what I suggest you to do:

- Miss lots of classes and/or come late many times
- Turn your assignments in late or don't hand them in at all

> Then, I will become very interested (too interested) in you and become quite interested in reading your mind...; otherwise, I am much too busy to do that and why would I want to intrude on your privacy in that way...?"

The above is one more example of my no longer *fleeing from my skills and from the omnipotent fantasies that can appear in their wake.*

Notes

1 Jean Charcot (1825–1893) was a French neurologist best known for his work on hypnosis and hysteria. His work greatly influenced the developing fields of neurology and psychology.

2 Freud talked in his autobiography of how, at the age of 9, he witnessed his father being bullied in the street by a Christian man who had ordered the father to come off the sidewalk and walk in the street. Freud had been shocked that his father had passively obeyed the bully. This observation is like the technical innovations of Wilhelm Reich (1948) who suggested that what the therapist should look for is not only what the patient says but also what he or she does not say. One may notice that my focus on the gratuitous remarks of the Presenter in the clinical presentation *flows directly from these observations of both clinicians*.

3 Kernberg, O. (1983), Personal Communication seminar in psychoanalytic technique.

4 I want to thank Kendra Terry for her permission to present this interaction.

5 Having had at least some indirect experience with one of these teachers (Reik was an important figure in my extended family; he has trained my aunt, that is, my mother's sister) as well as some direct experience with another (W.R. Bion 1978; Bion supervised my clinical cases in 1976), I can promise the following: In this book, I will strive to present the model that was elaborated and has evolved from Freud (1918) to Reich (1949) and from Reik (1948) to Bion (1962) and Winnicott (1960). I also promise that with a bit tweaking and elaborating, I will show how one can learn to do some version of their legacy in one's current work with psychodynamic therapy.

6 I am particularly grateful for the work of Kyle Arnold (2006) who has summarized Reik's work in a most thorough and thoughtful way.

7 Bion created a theory of thinking based on changing β-elements (unmetabolized psyche/soma/affective experience) into α-elements (thoughts that can be thought by the thinker). β-elements were seen as cognate to the underpinnings of the 'basic assumptions' identified in his work with groups: "the fundamental anxieties that underlie the basic assumption group resistances were originally thought of as *proto-mental phenomena...*forerunners of Bion's later concept of beta-elements." They were equally conceptual developments from his work on projective identification—from the "minutely split 'particles'." Bion saw as expelled in pathological projective identification by the psychotic, who would then go on to "lodge them in the angry, so-called bizarre objects by which he feels persecuted and controlled." For "these raw bits of experience he called beta-elements...to be actively handled and made use of by the mind they must, through what Bion calls alpha-functions, become alpha-elements." β-elements, α-elements, and α-function are elements that hypothesizes. He does not consider β-elements, α-elements, nor α-function to actually exist. The terms are instead tools for thinking about what is being observed. They are elements whose qualities remain unsaturated, meaning we cannot know the full extent or scope of their meaning, so they are intended as tools for thought rather than real things to be accepted at face value (1962, p. 3). Bion took for granted that the infant requires a mind to help it tolerate and organize experience. For Bion, thoughts exist prior to the development of an apparatus for thinking. The apparatus for thinking, the capacity to have thoughts "has to be called into existence to cope with thoughts". Thoughts exist prior to their realization. Thinking, the capacity to think the thoughts, which already exist, develops through another mind providing α-function (1962, p. 83)—through the *container's* role of maternal reverie. To learn from experience α-function must operate on the awareness of the emotional experience; α-elements are produced from the impressions of the experience; these are thus made storable and available for dream thoughts and for unconscious waking thinking... If there are only β-elements, which cannot be made unconscious, there can be no repression, suppression, or learning (Bion 1962, p. 8).

8 Schulman, M.A. (1982). Intelligence and Adaptation: An Integration of Psychoanalytic and Piagetian Developmental Psychology. Epistemology aims to answer questions such as "What do we know?" "What does it mean to say that we know something? "What makes justified beliefs justified?" and "How do we know that we know?" *Encyclopedia Britannica (June 2020)*. In my very rough estimation, I count that I have heard and supervised approximately 4 sessions/week for 30 weeks (15 weeks per semester) for each year that I have been a full-time teacher (this underestimates the supervision that I have done during summer months and the other cases that I have heard about at other times during a typical academic year). In this regard, I began teaching full time in the doctoral and postdoctoral programs at Adelphi University in 1974, and I wrote this in 2022. Thus, at the very least (it is probably significantly more), I have heard and supervised 5,760 sessions of psychotherapy. Of course, one might say and some friends who tease me have said this: *5,760 × 0 = 0, but if we assume that I have learned a bit of something from many of these cases, then I have had multiple opportunities to stock my mind with knowledge.*

References

Arnold, K. (2006) The need to express and the compulsion to confess; Reik's theory of symptom-formation. *Psychoanalytic Psychology, 23*(4), 738–753.

Billow, R. M., & Mendelsohn, R. (1990) The interviewer's presenting problem in the initial interview. *Bulletin of the Menninger Clinic, 54*(3), 391–414.

Bion, W. R. (1962) *Learning from experience.* London: Tavistock.

Bion, W. R. (1977) C f, Personal Communication, In R. Mendelsohn (Ed.), Critical factors in short-term psychotherapy. *Bulletin of the Menninger Clinic, 1978, 42*(2), 133–149.

Breuer, J., & Freud, S. (1896) Preliminary communication from studies on hysteria. In J. Strachey et al. (Trans.), *The Standard Edition of the Complete Psychological Works of Sigmund Freud, Volume II (1893–1895): Studies on Hysteria* (pp. 1–17). London: Hogarth.

Deutsch, H. (1942) Some forms of emotional disturbance and their relationship to schizophrenia. *The Psychoanalytic Quarterly, 11*(3), 301–321.

Fine, R. (1987) *The Development of Freud's Thought: From the Beginnings (1886–1900) Through Id Psychology (1900–1914) to Ego Psychology (1914–1939).* Lanham, MD: Rowman & Littlefield.

Freud, S. (1905) Fragments of an analysis of a case of hysteria. In J. Strachey et al. (Trans.), *The Standard Edition of the Complete Psychological Works of Sigmund Freud, Volume VII: ("Dora")* (pp. 1–122). London: Hogarth.

Freud, S. (1909) Notes upon a case of obsessional neurosis. In J. Strachey et al. (Trans.), *The Standard Edition of the Complete Psychological Works of Sigmund Freud, Volume X: Two Case Histories ("Little Hans" and the "Rat Man")* (pp. 151–318). London: Hogarth.

Freud, S. (1918) From the history of an infantile neurosis. In J. Strachey et al. (Trans.), *The Standard Edition of the Complete Psychological Works of Sigmund Freud, Volume XVII ("Wolf Man")* (pp. 7–122). London: Hogarth.

Freud, S. (1953) Fragment of an analysis of a case of hysteria. In J. Strachey (Ed. & Trans.), *The Standard Edition of the Complete Psychological Works of Sigmund Freud* (Vol. 7, pp. 7–122). London: Hogarth Press (Original work published 1905).

Freud, S. (1957) Mourning and melancholia. In J. Strachey (Ed. & Trans.), *The Standard Edition of the Complete Psychological Works of Sigmund Freud* (Vol. 14, pp. 237–258). London: Hogarth Press (Original work published 1917).

Haley, J. (1963) *Strategies of Psychotherapy.* New York: Grune & Stratton.

Haley, J. (1973) *Uncommon Therapy: The Psychiatric Techniques of Milton H. Erickson, M.D.* New York: W.W. Norton.

Kernberg, O. (1985) *Borderline Conditions and Pathological Narcissism.* New York: Jason Aronson.

Kohut, H. (2009) *The Restoration of the Self.* Chicago, IL: University of Chicago Press.

Mendelsohn, R. (2022) *Freudian Thought for the Contemporary Clinician: A Primer on Psychoanalytic Theory.* London: Routledge.

Mendelsohn, R., Bucci, W., & Chouhy, R. (1992) A survey of attitudes toward transference and countertransference. *Contemporary Psychoanalysis, 28*(2), 364–390.

Reich, W. (1933) *Character Analysis.* New York: Simon and Schuster.

Reich, W. (1949) *Character Analysis.* New York: Noonday Press.

Reik, T. (1932/1959) The unknown murderer. In J. Farrar (Ed.), *The Compulsion to Confess and the Need for Punishment* (pp. 3–173). New York: Farrar, Straus, and Cudahy.

Reik, T. (1948) *Listening with the Third Ear: The Inner Experience of a Psychoanalyst.* New York: Grove Press.

Reik, T. (1957) *Myth and Guilt: The Crime and Punishment of Mankind.* New York: George Braziller, Inc.

Reik, T. (1959b) The compulsion to confess. In J. Farrar (Ed.), *The Compulsion to Confess and the Need for Punishment* (pp. 176–356). New York: Farrar, Straus, and Cudahy (Original work published 1925).

Reik, T. (2003) A psychologist looks at love. In P. Roazen (Ed.), *Of Love and Lust* (pp. 1–640). New Brunswick, NJ: Transactions Publishers (Original work published 1944).

Rodman, F. R. (2003) *Winnicott: Life and Work.* London: Perseu.

Rogers, C. (1961) *On Becoming a Person: A Therapist's View of Psychotherapy.* London: Constable.

Strauss, B., Barber, J., & Castonguay, L. G. (Eds.) (2015) *Visions in psychotherapy research & practice: Reflections from the presidents of the society for psychotherapy research.* New York: Routledge Press

Shulman, M. A. (1982) Piagetian developmental psychology. *Psychoanalytic Review, 69*(3), 411–414.

Symington, J., & Symington, N. (1996) *The Clinical Thinking of Wilfred Bion* (pp. 12–13). London, UK: Routledge.

Winnicott, D. (1960) *The Maturational Processes and the Facilitating Environment.* New York: International Universities Press.

Winnicott, D. W. (1971) *Playing and Reality.* London: Tavistock.

Winnicott, D. W. (1964) *The Child, the Family, and the Outside World* (p. 17 and p. 44). London: Pelican Books.

Chapter 2

The Fourteen Clinical Processes Involved in My Approach to Case Formulation Including Countertransference, Inducement, Enactment, Projective Identification, and *Gratuitous Remarks*, and the Clinical Use of Many Processes Including Paradigmatic Techniques (and My Technical Use of My 'Sense of Humor')[1]

The terms that will be described in this chapter are the key concepts that I use in the formulation of clinical cases. Psychoanalytic/psychodynamic theory has changed and evolved over the last 120 years and so have the techniques related to it. That is, many of the techniques that were developed by Freud were based on his psychoanalytic theory of psychopathology and treatment. These included an emphasis on the psychotherapist's limited activity and limited responsiveness to the patient so that there would be a kind of interpersonal pull within the patient to produce unconscious material to be psychoanalyzed. What emerged starting in the late 1980s was the need to make the medium of psychodynamic treatment, supervision, and case formulation more symmetrical; this was one of the several changes that occurred as a result of the movement toward contemporary psycho-analytic ideas (Aron 1996), ideas about the structure of mind and about health, pathology, and treatment. And, as we've already begun to see in this book, in the Case Presentation format, the relationship between the teacher (Consultant) and supervisee (Presenter) is now considered by many to contain a considerable amount of data to be delineated and discussed by both members of the dyad. This is most accessible when it flows via an open discussion by both members of the Consultant/Presenter—*couple*. And, as you will see in this book, the *expert* should be very willing to discuss all aspects of this teacher/student situation with his/her student(s); and for obvious reasons, because of the issue of *timing, willing,* and *thoughtful about,* how to have this kind of conversation with one's own patients as well.

DOI: 10.4324/9781003375944-3

Psychoanalytic Techniques and Epistemology

In a very thoughtful paper, Lettieri (2005) revisits psychoanalytic/psychodynamic theory and its new relationship to the more interactive clinical approaches. He acknowledges that the psychic agencies of id, ego, and superego are now seen more as metaphors of psychological functions rather than as structures in their own right, as opposed to how they were understood in Post Freudian Ego Psychology (cf. Hartmann 1939). That is, these metaphors are now utilized to organize clinical observation and understand emotional conflict. Thus, the ego remains a valuable metaphor for the psychodynamic psychotherapist. What are the treatment implications of this? Lettieri cautions that—from the viewpoint of the ego as an organizing principal—if the psychoanalyst engages exclusively in natural and spontaneous relational exchanges (i.e., the more modern relational approach of psychoanalysis—Aron 1996), this may lessen interpersonal/intrapsychic tensions. One result of this is that it may also inhibit the patient's 'ego' from fully using the analytic process (and prevent the discovery of aspects of the patient's inner experience that would not otherwise appear and be known). Therefore, Lettieri suggests that the *neutrality* of the psychoanalyst provides *space* that not only protects the patient's individuality but also provides an opportunity for new aspects of the person to be discovered. Lettieri suggests to us that the art of the clinician is in *the balance that each dyad* achieves between optimal neutrality and optimal authenticity.

These observations focus on the therapy relationship, and they also highlight one difference between how soon one says something to one's patients (shares the *magic*, that is, the *psychological meaning*) as opposed to when one shares similar content with one's student/supervisee (or to the Presenter in a clinical presentation). In this regard, part of the issue of 'the clinician's magic' has to do with the timing of how soon a clinician reveals his/her thinking processes to the student versus to the patient.[2] That said, let me be as clear as I can about this issue regarding every clinical process: the general rule for me about when to reveal something to a person I am working with, in any context, is *the sooner the better.* However, as a rule of thumb, I find that one reveals earlier to other clinicians than one does with one's patients. Why is this? One reason for this is that if the clinician reveals something too early to one's patient, the patient may become upset/dysregulated, or in the worst-case scenario, the patient might conclude that their therapist is *crazy and/or destructive* (and, in a certain sense, because such an intervention often suggests a special/easy access to preconscious/unconscious material—the patient will be partly correct about the *crazy* part) (!). That is, if one means that *being crazy* is having an easier access to one's latent content, then *crazy* might be one conclusion to be drawn from a too-early intervention! This is why, for example, we use secondary processes as we awaken from a dream—the processes of secondary revision and secondary elaboration are employed to make rational meaning out of seemingly irrational dream images (cf Mendelsohn, 2022).[3]

Secondary revision suggests that one is revising history, that is, the image that you remember upon waking is being changed/revised on the spot because we can't reconcile it with the time, place, and person aspects of reality. With secondary elaboration, one is constantly and continually changing the images of a dream by adding features that weren't there before.

Here is what might be a typical example of the processes that occur when one is wakening from a dream:

> …So, first I thought that I was flying with my own wings. Then, I 'realized' that I wasn't flying without wings- I was viewing a friend who was flying his own plane. And, soon after I revised that: he wasn't actually flying his own plane— he was talking about going to flying school and I was jealous of this, etcetera…

That is, in secondary revision one changes (revises) the story, so that you are aligning it with the three spheres of time, place, and person, and in secondary elaboration, one is adding to the story—that is, adding features that are designed to further confuse/protect you, i.e., to keep you from the original latent material.

The goal of this revising and elaborating as we awaken from a dream is to make the latent content more disguised, so it is more acceptable to consciousness. If a person were to remember a very upsetting dream that was unfiltered, or a barely filtered dream—and thus, the manifest content of the dream was available, but the latent content was also available—this would be a dream that most people don't typically remember.

Here is an example of that kind of barely disguised dream.

The context of the telling of the dream

At the time that this occurred, I had just begun to add couple therapy to my clinical practice, and I got a call from a young woman. She wanted to see me with her boyfriend for a consultation. We worked out the time and I gave her directions to my office. At the appointed hour, I expected to see both, but when I opened the waiting room door, her boyfriend was there, but she was not. Where was she? She had driven them both to the session, he'd gotten out of the car, and she said to him: "You need help. I don't want to be with you anymore. You see the psychologist." Then she drove away. This is what he told me. He seemed like an emotionally damaged person; he could barely talk. Of course, he was now traumatized, but he also seemed quite odd, independent of this. Then, during the session he said, "I had a dream last night." He had known that he was going to have a session with a psychologist the next day, so I call such dreams "a transference dream" (his upcoming meeting with me influenced the dream).

Here is the Dream

Pt.:   "…I was walking in the woods and my foot knocked into a canvas bag. I opened the bag and there was a dead body. I realized I had to hide the evidence. So I ate it (the body)"

That was the dream. There was no elaboration. Hearing this dream was upsetting to me. I thought to myself: *Holy XXX, he's not supposed to remember dreams like this.* In other words, the latent content was barely filtered/barely hidden from consciousness. Thinking quickly, here's what I said:

Me: "What an interesting dream. I'll bet you're the kind of person who eats yourself up alive when you're upset."

Pt.:   "That's right," he said, showing some sign of relief.

We spent the rest of the session discussing how he was too hard on himself; he felt he could never get things right. At the end of the session, I asked if he wanted to return. He said he couldn't afford to see me alone: he and his girlfriend had been planning to share the cost. I gave him a list of clinics to apply for treatment, and I also asked him to contact me after he'd arranged to do this. Fortunately (one has little control over this), he did call after he made an appointment at a recommended facility.

I want you to understand that this dream was unusual because the dream work did not adequately disguise the manifest content from the latent content. I also want to tell you what *I think* the dream was about. I think the dream represented that he believed he killed every meaningful relationship through his inadequacy, hate, envy, and greed (eat) and that he had to hide the evidence of another failed relationship. I think he saw/sensed the breakup coming. I have no proof of the accuracy of my understanding of the dream and only could have had this (at least partially) confirmed had he and I worked on the dream together. However, I believe that this is an example of why Freud called dreams "the royal road to the unconscious" (cf, Mendelsohn 2022).

To continue, why would a clinician be concerned if a person presents with such an unfiltered dream. If the dreamer is a clinician with some training in working with latent material, then the clinician has, over time, developed a kind of *space* to put such content inside of themselves, to examine it, understand it, and work with some secondary (i.e., so-called higher level) defenses. If not, such content will probably be very unnerving and dysregulating even to the clinician!

In this regard, as I have suggested previously, if one has worked with acutely psychotic persons in a hospital setting, then one often hears barely disguised (or not at all disguised) latent content. In my earliest training in hospitals (in the 1960s), I was taught to say to an agitated psychotic patient "*inside is outside and outside is inside*"; this comment was often quite helpful before some of the powerful antipsychotic medications because the patient would feel *understood* and thus more connected to a human being as opposed to his/her feeling that they were not quite part of the human species. This is one of several reasons that I suggest to clinical students that during their training, they get as much experience as they can in inpatient settings (and in outpatient facilities connected to inpatient settings) no matter what their ultimate plans are to work and practice clinically.

Finally, some of my colleagues and friends might disagree about whether I should have shared my experience of this dream with this patient at the time I heard it (I can only imagine the spirited argument with the late Lew Aron (1996)[4] and I might have had!). However, I suggest to you that in certain clinical situations (where the issue is about the timing of the clinician's comments), there is an adage that one needs to modify:

"...Strike While the Iron is Hot..." is on occasion best if it becomes: "...Strike While the Iron Is Cold..."

(cf. McWilliams, 1996)[5,6,7]

Definitions of Fourteen Clinical Processes Involved in Case Formulation

As I suggested above, the issues raised here have led me to the following (Fourteen) Definitions of Clinical Process. In this regard, it is important to emphasize that I believe all these processes are clinically relevant to both the patient/therapist relationship and the presenter/consultant relationship.

1 *Gratuitous Remarks*: Freud expanded his understanding of the unconscious that he had presented in *The Interpretation of Dreams* in two other works: *The Psychopathology of Everyday Life* (1901) and *Jokes and their Relation to the Unconscious* (1905). In *The Interpretation of Dreams*, Freud suggested that the unconscious of the dreamer contains infantile, wish-gratifying memories. In *Three Essays on a Theory of Sexuality*, Freud explored the nature of these infantile memories, suggesting that they consist of pleasurable desires developed in infancy and early childhood which center on the stimulation of bodily zones, each of which is required for human adaptation and survival. Problems in this development lead to neurosis. Fixations on one's bodily zones are in the mind, to prepare one for the *adult* pleasurable sensations of sexual union. This will result in procreation and the continuation of our species. The model of sexual development is designed so that one will someday choose a member of the opposite sex with whom to procreate. Not *all* humans need to have orgasm as their *aim* and to have an opposite sex partner as their *object*, with procreation as their *goal*. But, Freud suggests, there is a relationship between this sexual development and neurosis. In *The Psychopathology of Everyday Life* and in *Jokes and Their Relation to the Unconscious*, Freud continued to extend his understanding of the unconscious mind. He did so using the insights that he had gained from the psychoanalysis of neurotic patients. Starting with the observation that neurosis is an unconscious defense against intolerable experience, Freud now looked at a variety of normal phenomena, such as slips of the tongue, which had previously been thought to be accidental, and jokes, where he demonstrated that joke telling; like dreaming, neurotic symptoms and *Freudian slips* all follow an orderly process where there is a release, or a blocking (repression), of thoughts and emotions followed by a failure of the repression. However, in these phenomena, the failure of repression is temporary and the interference with the person's functioning is minor and brief.

In a similar fashion, throughout this book, I have labeled the unusual and/or out-of-place comments made by the presenter in his/her presentation: "gratuitous remarks, but in fact, as I always explain after, these remarks are always 'small gifts'." This is my real point; in the setting of the presentation of clinical material, they are gifts that one can use to 'decode' the Presenter's preconscious transactions as they emerge:

> that is why - after a gratuitous remark - I wait for the Presenter to continue their presentation before Intervene and either ask more questions or make a comment. These preconscious transactions always do emerge...even when the Presenter doesn't want them to emerge.

The translation of the metaphor(s) that appears out of these comments is an important way to understand and decode the hidden meaning of an enactment, that is, of an act or behavior that occurs in a therapy typically as an attempt to work through a person's traumatic childhood. We will see many of these enactments and their translations throughout this book.

2 **Countertransference:** The notion of countertransference has undergone considerable transformation and elaboration since Freud first introduced it in his 1,910 lectures to the 'Second Psychoanalytic Congress' of 1914. At that time, Freud restricted the concept to the influence that the patient's transferences may have on the analyst's unconscious feelings. Cautioning particularly that the analyst's reactions to the patient's erotic feelings might impair the analyst's objectivity, Freud's view of countertransference emphasized its possible dangers (Mendelsohn et al. 1992). Yet, countertransference as it was originally narrowly defined is only one type of emotional reaction that an analyst can have to a patient. In the 1940s, Freud's narrow definition was challenged by several writers (Racker 1949; Winnicott 1949; Heimann 1950; Little 1951, 1960; Tower 1956). These authors and others suggested that such reactions as the analyst's own transferences, identifications, and realistic reactions might all be included under the rubric of countertransference. An analyst might therefore respond to a patient by identifying with the patient or might experience the patient as an extension of the analyst's self. Such writers as Bion (1963) suggested that responses are deposited in the analyst's psyche by the patient through projective identification, and thus, the analyst can even become the container of the patient's wishes. As Fromm-Reichmann (1950) suggested, an analyst will also respond to a patient by having realistic reactions, perhaps even powerful emotional reactions, to the patient's actual characteristics and behavior. Are such responses as these to be considered counter-transferential, even though they may be conscious? Can they be used to help the analyst better understand the patient? In fact, currently, psychodynamic therapists welcome countertransference responses as clues to the patient's problems. Sandler et al. (1970) summarized the various meanings of countertransference in the literature: (1) the resistance of the analyst resulting from the activation of unresolved conflicts by

the patient's material; (2) the analyst's transference; (3) the analyst's characteristics of personality reflected in his or her work, which may or may not cause difficulties in the treatment process; (4) the totality of the analyst's unconscious attitudes toward his/her patients; (5) the analyst's 'blind spots'; (6) the analyst's conscious and unconscious reactions to the patient's transference; and (7) the 'normal' or appropriate emotional response of the analyst to his/her patient.

In a further advance, Racker (1968) differentiated between two categories of countertransference: *concordant* and *complementary*. The former refers to the therapist's empathic response to what the patient had felt in relation to an early object, while the latter is the therapist's unempathic response to what that object had felt toward the patient as a child. The Presenter who feels complementary countertransference toward the patient to be presented may react like a condemning parent toward that patient—thereby colluding with the patient in his/her bid to remain ill, while the Presenter in a concordant countertransference may induce sympathetic responses in the Consultant and the audience as the Presenter acts in the presentation in ways that are like the way the patient suffered in childhood. In sum, currently, many psychoanalytic therapists conceptualize countertransference as the use of the psychoanalyst's self-reactions and see this as a powerful therapeutic tool for both understanding and treating the patient (Mendelsohn et al. 1992). As you will soon see, I see these reactions as important clues to the deeper/preconscious interactions that are also occurring during the clinical presentation. These interactions can be vital pieces of data that help us to decode the deeper meanings of the clinical case.

3 **Complementary countertransference: (also, see above)** The therapist feels like a patient's early object relation. For example, in complement to the patient's early feelings of awkwardness in the presence of an autocratic father, in complementary countertransference, the therapist begins to feel and even begins to act like the patient's autocratic father. Or, as another example, the couple therapist who feels complementary countertransference toward one member may react like a condemning parent toward that member, thereby taking sides in the couple's fight and colluding with the couple in their bid to remain ill and perpetuate their repetitive bickering.

4 **Concordant countertransference: (also, see above)** The therapist feels what it must have been like to be the patient as a child. For example, the therapist begins to feel awkward and uncomfortable, the way that the patient felt when in the presence of his/her autocratic father.

5 **Enactment:** While it has been used in a colloquial and rather imprecise way for some time, the term *enactment* emerged more clearly in psychoanalytic literature during the 1980s. It can also be found in a chapter subheading in Ogden (1982). Its definition is still subject to controversy, and some use the term as a substitute for 'acting out,' due to the conceptual confusion and pejorative way in which this latter term has been used. In the most severe cases, the psychoanalyst's capacity is compromised, causing him/her to cross the boundaries of analytical treatment. The difference between this versus 'acting out' lies in the fact that

in the latter, the analyst is not included, participating only as an observer of the patient's actions. However, in an enactment, the psychoanalyst contributes subject to his/her own transferences and blind spots, being led by the relationship instead of accompanying it. In the other definition, enactment implies a positive strength in treatment. Once the analyst has understood it, he/she separates his or her own conflictive contribution from that of the patient, thus making the event useful to the progress of the treatment. It is in this way that enactments, induced via projective identification, can help to provide both the therapist and the supervisor with new understanding that can help to produce positive change in the patient. The process of unraveling the psychological meaning of all of this and of putting the meaning in the context of a valuable learning experience (a learning process that includes a viable psychological theory of motivation and etiology, a technique, and a theory of technique and the formulation of a preliminary treatment plan for the case) is what I plan to teach you in this book. I will do so by describing a theory of clinical communication that includes both the manifest and latent content of patient/therapist and consultant/presenter interactions. I will highlight my points by including vignettes from my many years of being a practicing clinician, a teacher of clinical process, and a clinical supervisor. However, it is important to state that I am not the first person to have approached this topic in this way, and I owe a debt of gratitude to those psychoanalysts/psychodynamic psychotherapists who have worked within the paradigm of the *mutual enactments* that occur within the clinician and his/her patient. Most notable here is the work of Levinson (1972, 1983). For Levenson, it was impossible not to interact with the patient, and the therapeutic power of psychoanalytic therapy is derived from the clinician's ability to step back from interactive embroilment, the mutual enactment, and to reflect with the patient on those enactments to which it led, that is, to reflect with the patient on what each was doing to, and with, the other. Invariably, Levenson found, the therapist/ patient interaction was a recreation of patterns of experience that typified the patient's early family relationships. Further, since the Consultant and Presenter are not in the room with the patient during the clinical presentation, their dyad is operating at a more removed level of abstraction. This can enable them to see things that the clinician/presenter alone cannot see during the session.

Here Is an Example of an Enactment[5]

Many years ago, a woman came to see me for psychodynamic therapy; she was a college professor, and I began to work with her two times per week. She was a very interesting person. I was a young man beginning my clinical practice, and I really liked her, she was in her 50s, and in our first meeting, she told me the following story:

   This woman had thought that she had a good marriage. One night nearing their 25th anniversary, she and her husband made passionate love, but the following morning her husband served her with a subpoena: he was filing for divorce. She was devastated.

We began the therapy and (I thought) we were working on her need to mourn the loss of her marriage (you will see that—in an odd way—we were). Therapy was going along swimmingly as far as I could see. Then, in what seemed to me to come out of nowhere, she came to a session and said:

	"I've made a decision; I'm going to see *the other one*."
I said:	"What other one?"
She said,	"I'm also seeing another therapist, at the same time that I have been seeing *you*."
	"Oh!" I replied "Well (*attempting to regain what little composure I could*), can I ask you a few questions? Is the other therapist female?"
Patient:	"Yes."
Me:	"And, she knows that you are working with me, but I didn't know about her?"
Patient:	"Yes."
Me:	"Had she suggested that you tell me?"
Patient:	"Well... no."
Me:	"So, I guess I was just served the subpoena." 1
Patient:	(*laughs at my comment*) "I really am appreciative of your understanding, and despite this, you've helped me a lot."

Then, she left, never to return.

Please notice that I never asked the patient anything about her own feelings, her thoughts, or about her decision, as I thought that any patient has the right to leave any therapist whenever they want to. My concern with this person, and with others where something like this has happened, is not *when* the person leaves, but *how* they leave.

Also, I thought that the other therapist's behavior was unconscionable, but I felt that any attempt to tell the patient this would not be helpful to her. What was being enacted in this vignette?

I believe that this woman needed to hurt and abandon *someone* in order to express the trauma of her having been unceremoniously *dumped* by her husband. That is, she *dumped me*. However, equally interesting in this example is the following question: what was the *other* (female) therapist enacting? I will never know, but I did have some speculations at the time; I will not share those speculations here, as they were at least in part coming from my own impotent rage. However, I will say that my use of humor in responding to this patient was an example of what is called a Paradigmatic Technique (also see # 12 below).

Paradigmatic techniques are the technical innovations used in the context of modern psychoanalysis (Nelson 1981; Sherman 1981; Spotnitz 1986, 2004). As the reader is by now aware, I use humor quite a bit to offer both interpretations and other similar comments—in my attempt to convey meaning to my patients.

6 Humor and Psychotherapeutic Interventions:[8] Freud (1927) recognized that there are benign, loving aspects of the self-superego relationship when he studied the dynamics of humor. And, as Bader (1993) suggests, although there is a tendency for psychoanalysts to frown on the use of humor as a technique, moments of humor can often be precious to the patient. The appropriate cautions about *using* the patient or enacting various conflicts around aggression, sexuality, narcissism, etc. can sometimes be taken to mean that humor in the analyst is always counterproductive. Recently, however, there has been an increased interest in examining all of the psychoanalyst's emotional reactions and non-interpretive behaviors in his or her work in order to find a place for such phenomena in our theory of technique. Bader presents two clinical vignettes. In the first case, psychoanalytic work was at an impasse because of deeply entrenched resistances that took the form of the patient's relentless dissatisfaction with the analysis and constant accusatory and self-accusatory recriminations. The analyst, after several consultations, changed his style and began actively using humor in the treatment. The patient responded with an increased ability to psychoanalyze himself and the interaction with the analyst, primarily because of identificatory processes and because the analyst's humor disconfirmed traumatic expectations. In the second case, the patient felt that neurotic fantasies had been traumatically confirmed in a previous analysis. The author's use of humor enabled the patient to feel stronger, both in his relationships and in the analysis, where he was increasingly able to face difficult material. As Bader suggests, the analyst's technique is often taken by the patient as an expression of the former's internal mental state and, as such, can confirm or disconfirm certain pathological expectations, fantasies, and beliefs. In some patients who have been traumatically affected by parents who consistently blamed their children for their own narcissistic injuries and depression, the experience of an analytic technique that is emotionally restrained, flat, or too affectively 'neutral' can reinforce symptoms and can be refractory to interpretation. In these cases, there can be some advantages to the analyst deliberately allowing himself or herself to interact humorously with the patient.

Here Is an Example of My Use of Humor in an Impossible Marital Interaction Concerning a Marital Couple's Constant Battle over Sex

The man in this case had been a shy and inhibited boy; the youngest of three boys and the combination of his shyness and his two older brothers' boyish *horsing around* left him feeling unprotected by his parents, and awkward and reticent. This continued into his adulthood, and when he met and fell in love with a young woman, she lamented that she had proposed marriage to him because: "… it would not have happened otherwise…" After ten years and two young children, they came to couple therapy because of a conflict over sex. He claimed that she continually rejected him, and she claimed that by the time he completed his nightly rituals, and the kids were put to bed, she was too exhausted to make love. We worked for a while on possible practical solutions for this…but try as they might; he always approaches her late and she always reluctantly turned him down or complied but resented him the entire (exhausted) next day. I pointed out that he now had his wife bullying him and depriving him of love the way his brothers and parents had done. They seemed to be doing a little better with this for a few weeks, until they arrived at a session, and she told me the following story: they had gone to an early dinner on Saturday night, came home; he paid the babysitter, and she went up to *slip into something more comfortable and intimate.* She doesn't remember how long it was before she fell asleep (he later acknowledged that he had begun to watch a TV show and didn't come up for 2 hours!). When he did come up, he found her sleeping and he soon fell asleep himself. At about 4 am, the wife woke up to someone poking on her left leg. She found her husband sitting at the edge of their bed; as she opened her eyes, she heard him say: "*I guess that we're never going to have sex again...*"

Before she could tell the rest of the story, I turned to her, and I said the following:

...That really turns me on...how about you?

Immediately, they both began laughing and, while laughing, this man also acknowledged that he was aware of the deeper meaning of what I had just said. He also acknowledged that the joke shocked him into recognizing how self-defeating he was acting. This is an example of my use of humor via a paradigmatic comment to move the therapy to a place of increased meaning.

7 **Interpretation:** In a typical interpretation, historical metaphors are suggested. The psychotherapist gives his or her 'best guess' as to what the person's experience with primary objects must have been that would have helped to develop a particular kind of dynamic. In individual psychotherapy, interpretations are typically offered in relation to transference, resistance, and defenses. For another example, in couple therapy, interpretations of the marital style are also possible not only in relation to the therapist but also in relation to how the person responds to his/ her partner—and how each of them responds to the inner couple itself. As Rutan (2014) suggests, interpretations have three components: (1) emotional impact, (2) cognitive impact, and (3) timing. Because of the volatile nature of certain patient/ therapist relations, it is sometimes best to "strike while the iron is cold," because until the affect is manageable, the patient may be unable to hear you.

Kinds of Interpretations

a "Presenter and Patient's Relationship": In psychodynamic group psychotherapy (Rutan 2014), one kind of interpretation is called a group-as-a-whole interpretation. Novakovic (2016) used concept of the group mentality and likened it to Klein's (1946) idea of the internal couple to suggest that the notion of a *couple* as an unconscious idea that exists in the mind of both members of the couple and influences the way they treat each other, and perhaps even how they are treated by others (cf. Mendelsohn 2017). In this way, one suggests that the *couple* or, for our purposes, the patient/therapist dyad are greater than the sum of their parts. This same way of conceptualizing a clinical relationship can help us to deepen our understanding in the case formulation presentation.

When one makes a 'patient/therapist relationship-as-a-whole' interpretation, euphemisms are often employed.

Here is an example of a typical interpretative comment:

"I think you're wondering if your relationship with this patient can tolerate this." Here the term: "the relationship" serves as a euphemism for the unconscious representation of the therapist/patient-as-a-whole.

There are two kinds of 'therapist/patient relationship-as-a-whole' interpretations used in case formulation. (1) Consultant focused: These comments are focused on the transference to the Consultant and how he or she is being responded to by the internal 'couple in the mind of the therapist/Presenter.' (2) Presenter/patient focused: These comments focus only on the Presenter/patient aspect of the relationship—not on each individual member.

As we have seen above, the Presenter can have transference reactions not just to their patient but also toward the relationship between themselves and their patient. They can also have transferences to their relationship with the Consultant (one such transference might be as an *omnipotent savior* while another might be *as an interfering critical authority*). Presenter/Consultant-as-a-whole phenomenon can be evident, and they are part of what enriches the Presenter's (and the observers'/audiences') understanding of each other. When this *couple* can think in this way and apply what they have learned, the Presenter will be more aware of being able to engage not only in self-care but also in patient/therapist care. In fact, during a presentation, I found myself saying: "This supportive part of our relationship needs to be even more nurtured right now."

b Patient/Presenter interpretations: An interpretation of the Presenter can also be powerful because the Presenter may be able to hear something from the Consultant that the patient has been trying to tell them, but it has been harder for him/her to hear from the patient. Conversely, the containing presence of the Consultant may make it possible for the Presenter to hear something from the Consultant that he/she was unable to hear before.

c Individual interpretations: As I have indicated above, these are often historical metaphors made by the Consultant, kind of like 'best guesses' about what the '*patient being presented*' experience with his or her primary objects might have been. Freud (1912) called this process reconstruction, that is, using the current material to reconstruct the patient's past.

It should also be noted that any interpretation to any one individual within this mix, that is, to the Presenter/About the Patient/To the Audience/About the Patient/To the Consultant/About the Patient/To the Audience about the Presenter/To the

Audience about the Consultant, also impacts every other person in the room. And further, one technique a consultant may use when the Presenter is resistant to hearing something from the Consultant is to make an interpretation to other members of the assembled.

Here Is an Example

"You know that X (the patient) often seems to get very hurt when this Presenter is asking her historical questions and not staying in the 'here' and 'now'; the origin of this, I'm guessing, is because of how this patient felt so rejected by her father…"

Here the Consultant's comments are being employed to help the Presenter become more emphatic to his patient's resistance.

8   **Inducement:** The concept of induced countertransference has a long history. It first appeared in a letter from Ferenczi to Freud on February 7, 1911: "Besides monitoring the countertransference, one must therefore also pay heed to this 'being induced' by the patients (perhaps it is only a question here of a form of countertransference)". Sandler (1987) describes how pathological character induces or compels the psychoanalyst into certain roles or to experience specific affects that potentially provide the most immediate access to the patient's inner representational world. The notions of role responsiveness and inducement as they pertain to countertransference reactions have been viewed as a critical medium for grasping the patient's inner world with a yield of achieving contact with the patient's walled-off needs. In this regard, Grinberg (1972) talks about certain behavior of the patient that 'induces' the analyst to act out. Thus, one undesirable result of the analysis of trauma is that the subject tends to involve his or her objects in the repetition of the traumatic event, inducing them to reproduce its destructive effects. This can also take place at the level of the relationship between psychoanalyst and patient and between couple and therapist and between the patient/therapist—Presenter and Consultant. Below, we will see many examples of the Inducement of powerful thoughts and feelings in the therapist/Presenter *from the patient*, which has led to an Enactment of the patient's major conflicts *by the Presenter to the Consultant (and audience) in the presentation.* In this regard, it is my contention that *Gratuitous Remarks,* Countertransference, Enactment, and Inducement are all aspects of the process of Projective Identification (see below).

9   **Omnipotence:** Omnipotence means perfect power. It is the power that is free from mere potentiality, and its range of activity is limited only by the '*Powerful Beings*' sovereign will.' Freud (1909, 1927, 1918) viewed a feeling of omnipotence as intrinsic to early childhood, and he considered that in the neurotic, the omnipotence that the patient ascribes to his/her thoughts and feelings is a relic of the megalomania of early childhood.

10   **Paradigmatic Techniques and My Sense of Humor:** As I said above, Bader (1993) and others suggest that there is a tendency for psychoanalysts to frown on the use of humor as a technique. Yet, moments of humor can often be precious to

the patient. The appropriate cautions about using the patient or enacting various conflicts around aggression, sexuality, narcissism, etc. can sometimes be taken to mean that humor in the clinician is always counterproductive. Recently, there has been an increased interest in examining all the analyst's emotional reactions and non-interpretive behaviors in his or her work to try to find a place for such phenomena in our theory of technique. The analyst's technique is often taken by the patient as an expression of the former's internal mental state and, as such, can confirm or disconfirm certain pathological expectations, fantasies, and beliefs. In some patients who have been traumatically affected by parents who consistently blamed their children for their own narcissistic injuries, depression, and disappointments, the experience of a clinical technique that is emotionally restrained, flat, or too affectively 'neutral' can reinforce symptoms and can be refractory to interpretation. In these cases, there can be some advantages to the analyst deliberately allowing himself or herself to interact humorously with the patient. Here is an example of the use of humor when a clinician/Presenter had been presenting a couple who were hopelessly deadlocked in a struggle and wanting (demanding) their therapist to tell them who was *right* and which one of them was *wrong*.[9]

The Truth Lies Somewhere in between

This joke describes how couples push and pull each other and the therapist, via projective identification and enactment, to take sides in their battle.

"...Dr. Schoenfeld Is the World's Greatest Couples Therapist..."

Dr. David Schoenfeld, the World's Greatest Couples Therapist, says a joke that I like to tell couples when the time is right: A woman is dragging a man into the doctor's office, while the man is yelling for her to let him go. Dr. Schoenfeld introduces himself and tells them to sit down. The woman, obviously distraught, says:

"Thank you for seeing us, doctor. We have been married for over 20 years, and I thought that we were happy, but last night, he told me that he is in love with another woman. I can't eat, can't sleep. I'll do anything to save this marriage"

"Let me talk!" says the man. "I have never seen this woman before today. I am a waiter in the coffee shop on the first floor of this building. I just served her a cup of coffee, asked if she wanted anything else. She didn't answer, but instead she grabbed my wrist and dragged me all the way up here to tell you this ridiculous story."

Dr. Schoenfeld strokes his beard and says, "Ah, I think I know your problem. The truth lies somewhere in the middle."

Of course, in this (fictional) example, *there can be no middle and any suggestion of such would be ridiculous!*

Throughout this book, I will continue to present examples that include both a wry wit and a sharp sense of humor to convey—at times, quite painful, emotional experiences. That said, an improper (*out of sync*) humorous comment might be experienced by the patient as insensitive and even as sadistic. That is one more reason that a therapist needs to be as aware of his/her own emotional relationship with the patient as the patient's relationship is with them. We will soon talk about the *power of words* to convey/uncover and produce meaning within the clinical frame.

This is true in the relationship between the therapist and the patient, the therapist and the supervisor, and the Presenter and the Consultant.

11 **Projective Identification:** Projective identification is a term first introduced by the child psychoanalyst Melanie Klein (1946). It refers to a psychological process in which a person strives for emotional balance by engaging in a particular kind of projection. Projective identification differs from simple projection in that it is a kind of 'interpersonal self-fulfilling prophesy' whereby one individual relates to another in such a way that the other person alters their behavior to make the projector's belief(s) true. However, it is understood that this induction of a self-fulfilling prophecy is unconscious rather than overt. The very nature of unconscious inducement makes this kind of communication more powerful and potentially more malignant. As we see repeatedly in this book, projective identification is a common mode of communication between intimates, and therefore, it is not necessarily seen only in the most-disturbed, e.g., borderline and psychotic, populations. Projective-identificatory communications are attempts on the part of each member of any kind of *pair* (e.g., patient/therapist and Presenter/Consultant) to influence the other, that is, to incite the other member into feeling/action states. Projective identification may be indicative of borderline and other serious psychopathology in one or both members of a couple when it appears as a part of a complex of other primitive defenses, such as omnipotent control, but it is not necessarily pathological in every case. Traditionally, projective identification had been understood as a developmentally early and primitive psychological process and one of the more malevolent defense mechanisms (Klein 1946; Kernberg 1975; Ogden 1982). Yet, McWilliams (1996) suggests that while projective identification can still be seen as a pathological defense, ironically it can also be thought to be the psychological process out of which more mature psychological functions, such as empathy and intuition, are formed. In her book *Psychoanalytic Diagnosis* (1994), McWilliams points out that projective identification combines elements of projection (attributing one's own feelings, thoughts, and motives to others) and introjection (incorporating the feelings, motives, and thoughts of others). Thus, as has been suggested above, projective identification validates one's projections by making the projections real. There is also room in this conception of projective identification for the possibility that an individual employing the defense has seen and recognized something real—though latent and unconscious—in the other person, not merely made it come about. This recognition of the other's unconscious content is the common thread between projective identification and empathy. Throughout this book, I will be presenting examples of what, at first blush, might appear to be strange coincidences or, more unusual, special clinical abilities to find the hidden meaning in seemingly random clinical occurrences, that is, the so-called magic that my students have teased me about over the past 48 years. I will also demonstrate that this magic is nothing more than following the principles presented by Freud (1912) and his followers

(e.g., Reik 1948; Ferenczi 1993), that they are teachable, and, thus, that they are learnable. I contend that teaching and learning these processes can be done rather quickly and that there is less *magic* in these processes than hard work and continued practice in translating preconscious data into conscious metaphor.

To continue, considerable empirical data, garnered particularly by Beebe (2018), indexing the nonverbal matching behavior of partners, indicate that partners induce similar affective and subjective states through facial expression alone. Again, although this attunement to a mate is essential to making a shared life run smoothly, it is also what makes *all dyads* susceptible to projective identification and to confusion about boundaries between inside/outside.

12 **Resistance:** Menninger (1958) describes resistance as the process of forces within the patient that resists the psychoanalytic cure. The major resistance to the treatment is the patient's distorted thoughts and feelings about the therapist, crystalized in the transference.

13 **Transference:** Freud's first direct reference to the process of transference occurred in a footnote to the case of *Dora* (1905), when he mentioned that he had made an error with Dora's treatment by not working with her father-transference feelings to him. McWilliams (1996) suggests that Freud moved to a more interpersonal theory of treatment when he began to look more closely at his patient's transferences toward him, seeing them not as mere distortions to be explained away but as opportunities to provide the emotional context necessary for the healing that occurs in the psychoanalysis. These strong and oftentimes distorted feelings toward the psychoanalyst could be used as an analog for the distorted feelings the patient has toward his or her caretakers. These feelings have also been generalized to many other people in the patient's life and lead to inhibitions and other disturbances of function. For example, as this would apply in work with a couple, if a man felt undermined by his mother, he might be unable to distinguish his wife's motives (love and helpfulness) from his mother's motives (undermining, contemptuous, and critical).

14 **Working Through:** Working through is the process of generalizing an insight, interpretation, or other intervention so that the person understands and can apply this understanding to more and more of his/her behavior. As Menninger (1958) has suggested, it is very difficult for a person who has not studied unconscious functioning to understand the concepts and the meaning that are being introduced into the therapy. When that understanding begins to occur, the person will become more able to take the insights that he/she has learned and apply these insights to other, similar situations and circumstances.

A quick example of Working Through, from a couple's therapy, might be helpful:

Amy and James come to a couple therapy session, after a difficult previous session where they had explored James' discomfort with closeness. In this current meeting, they talk about a fight that seemed to have come out of nowhere, but soon James remembers that they had had a passionate evening the night before this fight, and he wonders if they were both tense because of that closeness. This leads the couple to talk about other times when one or both has found a way to start a fight after a period of closeness; they are reminded of the previous session, and they both talk about previous romantic relationships as well as each of their parents' marriages. Following this, they discuss ways that they can be more aware of this dynamic in their own relationship.

A Summary of the Major Theoretical Roots of My Approach to Case Formulation That Have Been Introduced above

Freud (1918) developed a very important clinical technique: talk therapy. This psychoanalytic technique is comprised of the following:

- Free association
- Detailed inquiry
- Reconstruction
- Interpretation, that is, the process where the therapist correlates the patient's reconstructions to his or her symptoms

Wilhelm Reich (1948) elaborated on Freud's insight that every neurotic disorder is a conflict between repressed instinctual demands and the repressing forces of the ego. However, he added that making conscious what had been unconscious needs to occur indirectly by eliminating the patient's resistance; this is the key to the resolution of the neurosis. The patient must first find out *that* he/she defends himself/herself, and then, *by what means* that he/she defends himself/herself, and only then, the patient can find *against what they are defending.*

Theodore Reik's (1948, 1959) observations suggest that humans have a powerful need to communicate our deepest parts to others. This observation lends support to my own theory of preconscious communication.

Winnicott (1960, 1971) considered that the "mother's technique of holding, of bathing, of feeding, everything she did for the baby, added up to the child's first idea of the mother," as well as fostering the ability to experience the body as the place where one securely lives. Extrapolating the concept of holding from mother to the family and to the outside world, Winnicott saw as key to healthy development "the continuation of reliable holding in terms of the ever-widening circle of family and school and social life" (1973, page...).

Bion's (1963) concept of maternal 'reverie' as the capacity to sense (and make sense of) what is going on inside the infant has been an important element in our current understanding of the patient/therapist conscious and preconscious transactions. "Reverie is an act of faith in unconscious process... essential to alpha-function." It is considered the equivalent of Winnicott's maternal preoccupation.

In the early 1960s (during the years of my doctoral studies), there were two dominant forces in clinical psychology training: post-Freudian Ego Psychology and Behavior Therapy Mendelsohn & Harmatz (1977). Both approaches were quite fixed and rigid in their approaches. Post-Freudian Ego Psychology would soon modify itself into several newer more flexible approaches: Self Psychology and Object Relations Theory (which would itself branch off into the field of Relational Psychoanalysis), while Behavior Therapy would later branch off into Cognitive Behavior Therapy (and one off-shoot of this is now Dialectical Behavioral Therapy).

The original forms of these therapies (post-Freudian Ego Psychology and Behavioral Therapy) seemed more connected to me because, having studied them together, I was struck that both had roots in the clinical technique of hypnosis—a treatment approach that I was also exposed to at several of my clinical placements. I was also led to the work of Milton Erickson (Haley 1973) and Jay Haley (1963). These brilliant clinicians understood the power of words in both the hypnotic state and the state of conscious wakefulness. The richness of their thinking, as well as its practical implications, opened up my eyes to a whole new way of understanding how humans communicate verbally to each other while often not fully recognizing the implications of their communications. You have already seen and will again observe this *in plain sight* as we continue to *decode* the preconscious symbols/metaphors of our patients/students/supervisees and Presenters.

Strategic Therapy is any type of therapy where the therapist initiates what happens during therapy and designs a particular approach for each problem. As Haley wrote in *Uncommon Therapy: The Psychiatric Techniques of Milton H. Erickson MD*: "Strategic therapy isn't a particular approach or theory, but a name for the types of therapy where the therapist takes a certain amount of responsibility for directly influencing people" (p. 17).[7]

Below is an illustration of the hidden power of words and phrases to convey preconscious meaning and to thereby influence the other:

VIGNETTE

Person A. is often quite provocative to Person B.; that is, Person A. 'attacks' Person B., while B. is *off guard* with unexpected, but mildly critical, comments always said in a 'cheerful tone.'

One day, Person B. decides that he/she has *had enough:*

Person B. encounters Person A. at the market. Person A. says: "Don't you ever get to the dry cleaners…that shirt is all rumpled…"

Person B. says (in a calm voice): "What do you mean?"

Person A. (a bit flustered) says: "You know…it's a mess…"

Person B. says (in the same calm voice): "I don't understand…"

Person A. becomes visibly agitated and says: "I've got to go…"

What has occurred here? Seemingly nothing much, but actually *a lot has occurred!*

What has happened is that up until this point, Person A. has counted on the use of a cheerful tone to be nasty and undermining of Person B. (since I'm writing the script here I want to add that in Person A.'s childhood, his/her father had a history of attacking this person but *wearing counterfeit tones and a phony sense of humor... and, if Person A. had complained to his father, he would be told that he was being "too sensitive..." a way to add further insult to the injury.* By matching Person A.'s *tone* but refusing to act as expected... that is by *not* being miffed and annoyed, Person B. has altered the script so that he or she has, in effect, said: "If you want to attack me you will have to do this openly and to my face...since I'm guessing that you don't want to be labeled a nasty jerk - you will probably run away like most cowards..."

In other words, while in this anecdote, the writer (me) is sympathetic to person A., having been tortured by his father during his childhood, I am not sympathetic to his attempt to do the same with Person B. now.

Here Is Another Phrase That Conveys More Meaning Than the Speaker May Know

Person A. is attempting to win an argument with Person B. by bullying and belittling. This has worked with Person B. in the past because Person B. had a bullying father and had been *trained in his/her childhood to give in and surrender—even when they knew that their argument was probably correct.* However, Person B. has now had some coaching from *Magic Bob.*

Person A.: "Listen, you don't know what you're talking about...yes, you went to school in engineering but I know more about engineering...even with my MBA education... than you ever will..."

Person B.: "I'm confused?"

Person A.: "Of course, you're confused...because you're an idiot...I said, you don't know what you're talking about ..."

Person B.: "What do you mean?"

Person A. (flustered): "I've got to go...you're an idiot (said with a weakened voice...)"

What Person A. does not realize in this interaction is that "I'm confused" is not a description of Person B.'s current state. It is an *accusation* that Person A. is confusing Person B. because Person A. is himself/herself *confused* and therefore Person A. is the *defective one.*

Here Is One Final Example to Demonstrate Again the Power of Words to Influence, Trigger and, Most Importantly, to Both Make Meaning and Change One's Perspective

A common phrase used quite a bit in our current social climate can be seen *in italics* within the following interchange:

Person A.: "We are very backed up with our job flow. Can you stay late at work for the rest of the week so we can move things along?"
Person B.: "...I'm not comfortable with that..."
Person A.: "Oh...oh...OK."

By using the above phrase "I'm not comfortable...," Person B. has now, in effect, made Person A. *responsible for his/her level of comfort.* If one follows the train of logic with this phrase, the first time Person A. accepts this *assignment of responsibility—he/she may not fully appreciate the implications of what it is that they are agreeing to, but a deal is a deal!*

In this regard, please keep in mind that I am describing this phrase and the possible meanings associated with it. I'm not suggesting whether it is being appropriately employed in any interaction. What I am suggesting is that words have power and meaning, the power to influence/encourage/discourage/seduce/reject/empower/control. And, further, when phrases are used by the clinician, with an understanding of both the conscious and the preconscious implications of their effects, these words and the phrases connected to them have power.

All of the above, in conjunction with all of the other examples that I am describing throughout this book, have led me to where I am today, the place of the so-called Special Clinical Powers that I have been my label in both my clinical treatment and my clinical supervision.

Billow and Mendelsohn (1990)

The final part of my journey to the present work occurred in the late 1980s/early 1990s when my colleague (Dr. Richard Billow) and I began to explore the complex processes of transference and countertransference that occur as early in a therapy, as in the initial interview. In *The Interviewer's Presenting Problems in the Initial Interview* (1990), we suggested that it is not only *the patient* who has presenting problems at a first interview but in fact the *interviewer* himself or herself has 'presenting problems' as well.

From this early work with Billow, I soon began to focus on the subtle and not so subtle processes that occur in the preconscious transactions between the therapist and his/her patient (Mendelsohn et al. 1992). This was the origin of the work that is often now labeled by my students and colleagues as the '*magic.*'

My Current Approach to Case Formulation

With the above, we can see the several models of psychotherapy that have influenced my approach to creating *magic*. In sum, I have been influenced in my thinking by several currents in psychotherapy, including hypnosis (M. Erickson), communication theory (Haley), Freudian psychoanalysis (Freud/Reich/Reik), psychoanalytic object—relations theory (Winnicott/Bion), relational psychoanalysis (Aron 1996), and psychodynamic individual/group and family psychotherapy (Billow/Mendelsohn).

Summary

Throughout this book, I demonstrate the processes observed in Case Formulation. This includes the processes of Transference and Countertransference, Inducement and Enactment, as well as the use of Paradigmatic Techniques and Humor. At the same time, I also demonstrate how our use of language is a valuable tool to understand both the Presenter and the Case Presentation. I also demonstrate that one result of more fully understanding the Presenter's reactions to his/her Case is that we may then more fully understand the Presenter's Case itself and perhaps understand it at a deeper level than the Presenter currently understands it himself/herself.

And, finally, as I have suggested, all the processes described above can also be seen to be informed by, and more closely understood via, examining the *preconscious process* of projective identification (see also Mendelsohn 2009, 2017, 2019, 2022).

Notes

1 I want to thank Roberta Karp for her help and encouragement regarding my approach to humor as a clinical technique.
2 The translation of a metaphor is one way to understand and decode the hidden meaning of an enactment, that is, of an act or behavior that occurs in a therapy typically as an attempt to work through a person's traumatic childhood. We will see many of these enactments and their translations throughout this book.
3 This example is taken from my book *Freudian Thought for the Contemporary Clinician* (Mendelsohn 2022).
4 Paradigmatic techniques are a technical innovation first suggested by Coleman Nelson (Spotnitz 1976, 2004; Coleman-Nelson 1981; Sherman 1981), who introduced the psychoanalytic model known as paradigmatic psychotherapy. In paradigmatic treatment, the psychoanalyst is understood to enact different roles that are induced by various ego states of the clinician. These techniques are seen as helpful with distrustful patients; the clinician joins the patient's system (i.e., their distrustful ideas) but also continues to support the patient's manifest negative feelings. When this is done empathically, the patient experiences that the clinician understands them. From this, a more positive transference can evolve; one result is the patient begins to question their distrustful ideas/beliefs.
5 Timing:
    When I teach psychodynamic psychotherapy to doctoral and postdoctoral students, they often ask me to talk about the most important component of psychotherapy

technique. My answer is to have one student role-play a scripted *interview* with me, but the 'interview' is the setup for a silly joke.

The Joke:

The student is to ask me, "I understand that you are the world's worst comedian."

And I will reply. Then the student is to ask me, "What is the secret of your success?" And I will reply again. Here it is:

Student: I understand that you are the world's worst comedian.

Me: That is correct. I am the world's worst comedian.

Student: What is the—

Me: Timing.

Clearly, in this example, my timing is totally off, and I have made my point with my joke. I believe that one secret of success in all clinical matters (therapy, formulation, and supervision) is one's *timing*.

BTW, I also understand that my *timing* has been part of my identification for much of my life. During late high school and college, I was a professional drummer working with several well-known performers. One of the greatest compliments that any musician can give a drummer is when they say:

"You're really *in the pocket*..."

This means that your timing is impeccable.

6 I want to thank Nancy McWilliams (1996) for this valuable idea.

7 Lew Aron was one of the founders of Relational Psychoanalysis (Aron 1996). This is a school of psychoanalysis that emphasizes the role of real and imagined relationships with others in both psychopathology and psychotherapy. Relational Psychoanalysis began in the 1980s as an attempt to focus on the detailed exploration of interpersonal interactions (interpersonal psychoanalysis) with ideas about the psychological importance of internalized relationships with other people (object relations theory).

8 Jay Douglas Haley (July 19, 1923 – February 13, 2007) was one of the founding figures of brief and family therapy in general and of the strategic model of psychotherapy, and he was one of the more accomplished teachers, clinical supervisors, and authors in this discipline. After a year spent in pursuit of a career as a playwright, he returned to California and received a BS in Library Science degree from the University of California at Berkeley and then a master's degree in Communication from Stanford University. While at Stanford, Haley met the anthropologist Gregory Bateson who invited him to join a communications research project that later became known as The Bateson Project, a collaboration that became one of the driving factors in the creation of family therapy and that published the single most important paper in the history of family therapy, "Towards a Theory of Schizophrenia." The central members of this project were Gregory Bateson, Donald deAvila, Jay Haley, John Weakland, and Bill Fry.

9 I have called the kind of couple who fight in front of their couple therapist while demanding that the therapist determine which one of them is *right* a *Sibling Couple* (Mendelsohn 2017).

References

Aron, L. (1996) *A Meeting of Minds: Mutuality in Psychoanalysis*. New York: Routledge.

Bader, M. (1993) The analyst's use of humor. *Psychoanalytic Quarterly, 62*, 23–50.

Beebe, B. (2018) Comment on micro analysis of multimodal communication in therapy: A case of relational trauma in parent-infant psychoanalytic psychotherapy. *Journal of Infant, Child, and Adolescent Psychotherapy, 17*(1), 1.

Bion, W. R. (1963) *Elements of Psychoanalysis*. New York: Basic Books.

Brabant, E., & Ernst Falzeder, G.-D. (Eds.) (1993). *The Correspondence of Sigmund Freud and Sándor Ferenczi 1908–1914*. Cambridge, MA: Harvard University Press.

Coleman-Nelson, M. (1981) The paradigmatic approach: A parallel development. *Modern Psychoanalysis*, *6*(1), 9–26 (Some forms of emotional disturbance and their relationship to schizophrenia. *The Psychoanalytic Quarterly*, *11*(3), 301–321).

Ferenczi, S. (1994) *Final Contributions to the Problems & Methods of Psycho-Analysis*. Sandor Ferenczi, H. Karnac Books. Cambridge, MA: Harvard University Press.

Frawley-O'Dea, M. G., & Sarnat, J. E. (2001) *The Supervisory Relationship: A Contemporary Psychodynamic Approach*. New York: Guilford Press (Dr. Frawley O'Dea is a graduate of our doctoral program).

Freud, S. (1905a) Fragments of an analysis of a case of hysteria. In J. Strachey et al. (Trans.), *The Standard Edition of the Complete Psychological Works of Sigmund Freud, Volume VII: ("Dora")* (pp. 1–122). London: Hogarth.

Freud, S. (1905b) *Three Essays on a Theory of Sexuality* (Standard Edition 7, pp. 151–318). London: Hogarth Press.

Freud, S. (1909) *Notes Upon A case of Obsessional Neurosis: Ratman* (Standard Edition 10, pp. 123–246). London: Hogarth Press.

Freud, S. (1912) Recommendations to physicians practising psycho-analysis. In *The Standard Edition of the Complete Psychological Works of Sigmund Freud, Volume XII* (pp. 109–120). London: Hogarth Press

Freud, S. (1914) Observations on transference love Standard Edition 12 157–171 London: Hogarth Press

Freud, S. (1927) Humour. *The Standard Edition of the Complete Psychological Works of Sigmund Freud, Volume 21, 159–165.*

Freud, S. (1918) From the history of an infantile neurosis. In J. Strachey et. al. (Trans.), *The Standard Edition of the Complete Psychological Works of Sigmund Freud* (pp. 7–122). *Volume XVII*. London: Hogarth Press.

Fromm-Reichmann, F. (1950) *Principles of Intensive Psychotherapy*. Chicago: University of Chicago Press.

Goodman, G. (2007) "I feel stupid and contagious": Quantitatively Based methods of assessing supervisee competence in clinical supervision. *Psychologist/Psychoanalyst, XXVII*(3). (pp. 1–26)

Grinberg, L. (1979) Countertransference and projective counteridentification. *Contemporary Psychoanalysis, 15*(2), 226–247.

Grotstein, J. S. (2005) 'Projective transidentification': An extension of the concept of projective identification. *The International Journal of Psychoanalysis, 86*(4), 1051–1069.

Haley, J. (1963) *Strategies of Psychotherapy*. New York: Grune & Stratton.

Haley, J. (1973) *Uncommon Therapy: The Psychiatric Techniques of Milton H. Erickson, M.D.* New York: W.W. Norton.

Hartmann, H. (1939) *Ego Psychology and the Problem of Adaptation*. New York: International Universities Press.

Heimann, P. (1950) On countertransference. *International Journal of Psychoanalysis, 31*, 81–84.

Kernberg, O. (1975) *Borderline Conditions and Pathological Narcissism*. New York: Jason Aronson.

Klein, M. (1946) "Notes on some schizoid mechanisms" *The International Journal of Psycho-Analysis, 27*, 99.

Levenson, E. (2005) *The Fallacy of Understanding and The Anatomy of Change*. London, UK: Routledge.

Lettieri, R. (2005) The ego revisited. *Psychoanalytic Psychology, 22*(3), 370–381.

Little, M. (1951) Countertransference and the patient's response to it *International Journal of Psychoanalysis, 32:32–40.*

McWilliams, N. (1996) *Psychoanalytic Diagnosis*. New York: Guilford Press.

Mendelsohn, R. (2009) The projective identifications of everyday life. *The Psychoanalytic Review, 96*(6), 871–894.Mendelsohn, R. (2017) *A Three-Factor Model of Couples Psychotherapy: Projective Identification, Level of Couple Object Relations, And Omnipotent Control*. Lexington, MA: Lexington Books/Rowman & Littlefield.

Mendelsohn, R. (2019) *Couple Dynamics Book By Novakovic, A*. London: Karnac Books (2016). Reviewed for the *International Journal of Group Psychotherapy.*

Mendelsohn, R. (2022) *Freudian Thought for the Contemporary Clinician*. London, UK: Routledge Press.Mendelsohn, R., Wilma B., & Chouhy, R. (1992) A survey of attitudes toward transference and countertransference. *Contemporary Psychoanalysis, 28*(2), 364–390.

Mendelsohn, R. & Harmatz, M. C. (1977) Length of stay and behavior patterns of hospitalized schizophrenics. *Psychiatric Services,* 28(4), 273–277.

Menninger, K. (1958) *Theory of Psychoanalytic Technique*. Basic Books.

Nelson, M.-C. (1981) The paradigmatic approach: A parallel development. *Modern Psychoanalysis, 6*(1), 9–26.

Novakovic, A. (2016) *Couple Dynamics*. London: Karnac Books.

Ogden, T. H. (1977) *Projective Identification and Psychotherapeutic Technique*. Jason Aronson, Incorporated. New York: Jason Aronson.

Racker, H. (1949) The Meanings and uses of countertransference. In H. Racker (Ed.), *1968 Transference and countertransference*. London: Hogarth Press.

Racker, H. (1968) *Transference and Countertransference*. London: Hogarth Press.

Reik, T. (1948) *Listening with the Third Ear*. New York: Grove.Rutan, K. J. S., Stone, W. N., & Shay, J. J. (2014) *Psychodynamic Group Psychotherapy (Fifth Edition)*. New York: Guilford Press.

Sandler, J. (1987) The concept of projective identification. *Bulletin of the Anna Freud Centre, 10*, 49.

Sandler, J., Holder, A., & Dare, C. (1970) Basic psychoanalytic concepts: Countertransference. *British Journal of Psychiatry, 117*, 83–88.

Sherman, M. H. (1981) Siding with the resistance in paradigmatic psychotherapy. *Modern Psychoanalysis, 6*(1), 47–64.

Spotnitz, H. (1976) *Psychotherapy of Preoedipal Conditions*. New York: Jason Aronson.

Spotnitz, H. (2004) *Modern Psychoanalysis of the Schizophrenic Patient: Theory of the Technique*. New York: YBK Publishers, Inc.

Tower, L. (1956) Countertransference. *Journal of the American Psychoanalytic Association, 4*, 224–255.

Winnicott, D. (1949) Hate in the countertransference. *International Journal of Psychoanalysis, 30*, 69–74.

Chapter 3

Early Clinical Examples of My *Knowing* (Without Consciously Knowing) What I *Unconsciously Knew*

In my training *and journey to become a psychologist*/psychoanalyst/psychody-namic psychotherapist/teacher/supervisor/Consultant, I had several experiences that, at the time, I did not understand, and therefore, I did not focus on them for too long, because they were quite confusing and some were also upsetting to me. It was only later in my professional life that these experiences began to make psychological sense. I will present a few of them now because the essence of my so-called magic is that I have taught myself how to *listen to a Presenter's clinical experiences, understand, decode, make meaning out of them and then translate that meaning to the other(s) in the session.* I learned this first by doing it with *myself.*

We have already seen examples of this work that I have done with others, and I have previously described what I believe to be the theoretical and technical reasons that I can do this (i.e., that I can *make meaning out of seemingly unexplainable/indecipherable* experiences). I now want to present three of my own unusual experiences that, at the time, I couldn't fully understand, but now, having honed my technique of the translation of preconscious processes into conscious processes, I can provide myself and the reader with a reasonable, meaningful, and coherent explanation for each of them.

Making Meaning Out of My Unusual Clinical Experiences

Here are the three experiences:

1 *My Illusion*

After receiving my doctorate in clinical psychology, I began my clinical psychology practice while I was teaching at a small college in a rural part of upstate New York. In the example below, I had rented office space in a professional office building that in another era had been a large old house. The first-floor living room/dining room and kitchen are now our administrative offices and bathrooms, while the several upstairs bedrooms were professional offices for the few psychologists, psychiatrists, and social workers practicing in this small town. My work directing our college clinic gave me access to all these practitioners, and I was soon encouraged to begin a small clinical practice. On one very dreary

DOI: 10.4324/9781003375944-4

late afternoon in December, I left my college offices and drove the short ride into town to meet for the first (and unbeknownst to me—only time) with a man in his early 30s. He was extremely athletic-looking and very handsome; he worked in his family's construction business. He was also missing his right arm and hand, so he quickly extended his left hand in greeting me. When I began to talk to him about his life, he quickly told me that his physician thought he should talk about the work accident that had occurred two years before and that had led to the amputation of his hand. This was the last time we talked about it during the meeting—as each time I attempted gently to return to the topic, he uttered dismissive comments such as: "what's done is done" and "talking won't bring me my hand back." Despite these comments, he presented as a reasonably upbeat person, and while he courteously thanked me for my *help,* he made it clear that he wouldn't be returning. This patient was my last session of that day. I wrote some notes and straightened out my desk and then I opened the closet door to get my coat, hat, and gloves. To remind the reader, the office was in an old house and my office room was an old, converted bedroom. Fastened to the closet door was a full-length mirror. As I opened the door, I was horrified because, for a split second, I could not see my entire right arm, including my right hand. "Well," I thought, "I have gone insane." I then reassured myself that what had occurred was a temporary illusion, not a hallucination, as it was a brief distortion of reality and not a full altering of reality. I also reasoned that this was like a kind of slip of the tongue or slip of the pen or mishearing of a word, what is commonly known as a '*Freudian Slip*'[1] Despite this attempt at self-soothing reassurance, what had happened was quite upsetting to me, and so on the way home, I tried to understand what had happened; why did I distort reality, and also, why was the patient so 'cheerful' during the session. After a nice meal and a soothing beverage, I helped myself to forget about the experience—only to remember it years later when I began my own training to become a psychoanalyst.

2 My Second Illusion

After a year at the upstate college, I realized that I wanted and needed more psychotherapy training, and I decided to return to the New York City area. In 1970, I returned to Long Island, and for several years, I was a Supervising Psychologist at a local hospital, while I also pursued postgraduate study in psychoanalysis at another Long Island institution, Adelphi University. At Adelphi, I completed two postdoctoral training programs: a four-year postgraduate program in Psychoanalysis and Psychotherapy and a three-year postgraduate program in Group Psychotherapy. In 1974, while a postdoctoral student, I accepted a position in Adelphi's clinical psychology doctoral program. I also began a practice in psychotherapy, and several colleagues began to refer people to me. One was a man in his 40s who was struggling with loss—the recent breakup of a girlfriend, the loss of a sister to cancer, and the serious illness of another sister, also struggling with the same kind of cancer. In this session (our only session), this patient seemed even-tempered, calm, and reasonable about his losses. This was surprising to me because the physician who had referred him to me was quite concerned about him.

Just as with the case above, I skillfully (I thought) attempted to bring the conversation back to loss and sadness, but to no avail. However, this time I didn't need to wait until the end of the session to experience something upsetting and weird in myself. As this man talked, I would look at his face, but I couldn't get the image out of my mind of a 'skull and crossbones' (i.e., a symbol of death). This time I clearly knew that it was only in my head, but it was still disconcerting. The session ended in a way not so different from the previous one that I mentioned above. That is, the patient left thanking me but saying that he had no interest in returning.

Several months later, I received a call from the referring physician who told me sadly that this patient had just been diagnosed with the same form of cancer that had taken the lives of his sisters and that he did not have very long to live.

What can we make of these two experiences? As we have seen above, Theodore Reik (1948) in his groundbreaking book *Listening with the Third Ear*[2] describes how psychoanalysts intuitively use their own unconscious minds to detect and decipher the unconscious wishes and fantasies of their patients. That is, according to Reik, psychoanalysts come to understand their patients best by examining their own unconscious intuitions about their patients. While Reik does not speak directly about this regarding the processes of supervision, in *Listening with the Third Ear,* he does comment about case formulation, and he develops a kind of *theory of listening*. Reik's theory of listening is organized around an emphasis on sequencing. He suggests that psychoanalytic listening has a natural sequence that begins with unconscious conjectures about a patient's dynamics and ends with conscious case formulations. Psychoanalytic conjectures crystallize out of the intersubjective, reciprocal illumination of the therapist and patient's unconscious minds. That is, psychotherapists understand their patients most deeply by becoming conscious of their own subjective reactions to their patients and by rigorously examining these reactions.

3   Here Is a Third Example:
As we're beginning to see, our unconscious system is very creative, and it is the source of important clinical information. I will now present a third example—an early memory (screen memory)3 that I recently had in a group therapy session with a group that I currently lead. This memory had me thinking (again) about the creative power of the unconscious and how it can be used clinically. It is an example where I used my own emotional reaction (by accessing an early memory that presented itself to me and illuminated my work in a therapy group that I had been leading):
Here is the context and then the memory:
During a group session, a memory returned to me that I hadn't thought about in many years. It is a wonderful example because it's so obvious when you hear it. The context is that in this group, there are two male group members who were talking about an old group—conflict between them (the conflict had occurred about a month before and I naively thought that it had been resolved). I said something about the resolution and, the next thing I knew, both men were enraged (first at each other, then at the group, and then, finally, at me). They

were both threatening to quit the group, even threatening violence against each other (given each man's history and psychological dynamics, violence, while not impossible, would be unlikely).

Here's the Memory

My mother is talking to a neighbor on the first (ground) floor of our apartment building (I'm about four years old). We're at the top of a long flight of stairs that leads down to the basement. The basement door is open because the basement is where the washers and the dryers are located, to clean tenants' clothes. I'm sitting on my tricycle, perched at the very edge of the stairway (I believe that my mother was just about to take me outside to ride my tricycle, but this could be a false elaboration of the memory).

I see nothing else in this memory, although the story I was later told was that the superintendent (caretaker) of the building saw me flying down the stairs and witnessed helplessly as I smacked into a basement wall and broke my nose in three places. I hadn't had this memory in a long time, but it came back to me when I was thinking about this book and thinking about what had happened in the therapy group. Early memories come back to us at various times, and it is as if the unconscious wants to remind us of something, teach us something. Maybe I had been feeling too arrogant, a bit too reckless in the group, or even feeling reckless about writing this book? In any case, this memory serves as a kind of warning to me: "stop flying around...get back to earth."

Perhaps it also says something about my mother's care/her inattention; it's a reminder to me: *Don't be as inattentive as she was on that day*. This comes home now that I have two young grandchildren and I am reminded again about how much attention a young child requires so that we can protect them from danger. Thus, this might also be a *rebuff* against myself:

> ...You didn't protect these group members from themselves and protect the group from the sudden explosion in the room, as expressed by these two members. That is, *by* being *inattentive, preoccupied, perhaps too interested in some other conversation(s), you failed in your protective function just as your mother had failed in hers!*

Words and Their Double Meaning as a Way of Deciphering the Preconscious

I will now return to a topic I discussed above (Chapter 2) about Paradigmatic Techniques and Humor. To remind the reader, these are technical innovations used in the context of the School of Modern Psychoanalysis (Spotnitz 1976, 2004; Nelson 1981; Sherman 1981). These techniques were first suggested by Coleman-Nelson (1956), who introduced the psychoanalytic model known as paradigmatic psychotherapy.

In paradigmatic treatment, "the analyst is conceived to enact different roles which are induced by various ego states of the analysand" (Sherman 1998, p. 486). Among those paradigmatic techniques having value is that of siding with the resistance. Spotnitz (2004) described this technique as a 'joining' procedure. As Sherman (1981) suggests, the technique is particularly helpful with patients who struggle with paranoid ideation, where the therapist is encouraged to not only join the 'system' (i.e., the paranoid system) but also continue to support the patient's 'manifest negative transference.' When this is done in an appropriate way, Sherman believes, the patient gets the feeling that the therapist truly understands them. And from this, a more positive transference evolves, with one result that the patient begins to question his/her distorted ideas. As Sherman states, "the patient spontaneously develops a self-critical faculty that in all likelihood has never been present to any effective degree" (Sherman 1981, p. 48).

The reader has already seen examples of my use of humor—often via a *paradigmatic* technique. An example of this is when I told a patient who informed me that she was suddenly quitting the therapy after she have been previously dumped via subpoena by her husband, and my response back to her was:

… Well, I guess I was just served with a subpoena…

I often use humor and sarcasm when dealing with impossible situations and/or when I want to make an important interpretation quickly and powerfully. Of course, as with any comments from the clinician—one needs to be aware of the possible (unanticipated) effects on the patient in order to avoid any needlessly insulting or hurtful comments that might cause a rupture in the therapeutic relationship.

In this regard, below are a series of words and/or phrases that convey a double meaning to the listener, and just as with the gratuitous remarks of a Presenter, I both listen to and employ these words and phrases when teaching my students my *unusual way of making meaning*. I do this to demonstrate that the use of a particular word or a phrase at a particular time conveys more than one meaning, and sometimes, the double meaning of the word or phrase conveys certain preconscious pulls to influence' the listener.

Here Is an Example

I once questioned a person who was attempting to sell me an insurance policy— later, he said that he wanted a *"brief moment of my time…"*

When I asked this man about the phrase (brief moment), he told me—with a bit of embarrassment—that he had been in a seminar at his insurance company during his training and they had given these salesmen in training a list of phrases to use in the in attempt to engage potential clients. As I said, he was intrigued, but also a bit embarrassed when I told him that this is the kind of phrase that has been used as a *prime* by hypnotherapists to induce a trance state (really a dissociative state) in patients who appeared resistant to trance induction (Erickson 1964).

In This Regard, Here Is a Historical Anecdote

My introduction to the processes of preconscious/unconscious communication and the importance of listening for latent clues from all members of the clinical enterprise (the patient, the therapist, the supervisor, the Presenter, and the Consultant) began early on in my training as a psychologist in the mid-1960s (but didn't crystalize for me until after I took training in psychoanalysis and psychoanalytic psychotherapy in the mid-1970s–mid-1980s). Ironically, not unlike Freud (I just put myself in good company!), these early experiences were highlighted when I was introduced to clinical hypnosis.

After receiving his MD degree from the University of Vienna in1881, in 1886 Freud went to France, to study with the famous neurologists, Charcot and Janet. After Freud left from studying in Paris, he began to collaborate with Dr. Josef Breuer, the most senior neurologist in the city of Vienna, who was working with hysterical patients. When they began their work, the field of the study of hysteria (neurosis) was in chaos, and the only people doing work of value were Charcot, Janet, and Breuer. Both Charcot and Janet's contribution was the use of hypnosis to both demonstrate and treat hysteria (each of these clinicians would put a patient under hypnosis and paralyze a limb, and then through the hypnotic trance, each was able to show that *with words* that the doctor could alter a somatic experience, that is, add or remove the paralysis). Following on the work of Charcot and Janet, Josef Breuer, from 1880 to 1882, treated a young woman, Anna O. (her real name was Bertha Pappenheim[3] and she later quipped that it was *she* who invented psychoanalysis; not Freud, because she believed that the most important part of her treatment with Breuer had *not* been the hypnosis process, itself, but instead it had been the *talking* that occurred before and after each trance state). In this regard, Freud practiced hypnosis into the late 1890s, but he gave up treating his patients with hypnosis. Freud began to realize that he didn't need to alter the patient's state of consciousness; if he simply asked the patient to say whatever came into his or her mind, without attempting to censor it, sooner or later the person would begin to come up with associations that led to memories. Those memories from childhood that emerged were understood as the opening to the person's entire unconscious psychology. Freud also gave up hypnosis because hypnosis pulls for people to be suggestible.[4]

My experience with hypnosis was a little less planned and a bit more dramatic.

In an incident that could never happen in this modern time, as a doctoral student I was externing at a hospital and the facility offered seminars as part of our training. One was a two-day intensive seminar on clinical hypnosis. I am sure that the reader will not be surprised to hear that even as a student I was a bit of a rebel, and when I heard the title of the seminar, I said loudly to the other assembled externs that this hypnosis seminar would probably be followed by a performance by a stage magician. However, I did not see the two Presenters behind my back. A few minutes after the seminar began, I began to feel very strange, and soon I was in what these presenters would later call a light trance. I was *hooked.* Although I never practiced exclusively as a hypnotherapist, over my many years of clinical practice

I have incorporated many of the lessons that I would later learn about the use of provisional/non-committal phrases, such as *perhaps* and *you might.*

This is what I mean.

A patient says:	"I could never be taught to *relax*, I'm too tense."
The clinician replies:	"OK but *perhaps* you'll feel a little differently as you breath in deeply…"

Keep in mind that in presenting these comments, I am not attempting to demonstrate hypnosis—only that certain words and phrases can induce/encourage feelings of suggestibility and thereby weaken resistances.

Here Are Some Others

"…I *just* have a question (I *only* have a question) …"

"…What do you mean?" (As I had said previously, this phrase forces the person to explain themselves, and there are times when a person might rather not say what it is they mean.)

"…I'm confused?" (This is not just a statement of fact—it is an accusation that the other person is confusing you!)

And here's a very common one that means much more than the hearer (and sometimes even the *teller*) realizes…

"…I'm not comfortable with that…" (If the *other* now apologizes for their request/comment, they are, in effect, agreeing that they are, as of now and perhaps forever, *responsible for this other person's level of comfort.*)

I have mentioned these phrases (and others) above, and I am highlighting them again (and the processes related to them) to demonstrate that the spoken word, when used thoughtfully in a clinical setting, can have much more power than the hearer, or perhaps even the speaker, consciously knows.

As we translate these processes by decoding the meaning of patient dreams and presenter communications in later chapters, I believe that you will see more clearly how this so-called magic really works.

Or, another way of saying all of this is:

…Perhaps the reader will soon find themselves agreeing with everything that I have been saying…

(Of course, the sentence above is a tongue-in-cheek-parody of what I just presented.)

My Training in Group Psychotherapy as a Further Confirmation of the Importance of Words to Convey Preconscious Processes

I mentioned above an early (screen) memory that returned to me recently in a group therapy session of a group that I currently lead. This memory had me thinking (again) about the creative power of the unconscious and how it can be used clinically. It is an example where I used my own emotional reaction to understand an interaction between me (the group leader) and the other members of the group. As I also mentioned, in 1970, I returned to New York and soon to postgraduate study in psychoanalysis and psychotherapy at Adelphi University. At Adelphi, I completed two postdoctoral training programs: a four-year postgraduate program in *Psychoanalysis* and *Psychotherapy* and a three-year postgraduate program in *Group Psychotherapy*, both at *The Derner School*. My training in Group Psychotherapy was a great influence on my way of listening and responding in the clinical interaction. It also helped me to listen to and even to *question everything I hear for its possible double meaning.* I remember the first time I realized that words, even rather simple words, can be used not only to communicate but also to obscure and block communication. With my supervisor, the late Dr. Bernard Frankel,[5] I was listening to an interaction in one of my groups, and a young woman was saying to a young man:

But I'm just curious about your relationship to XX (another group member).

Dr. Frankel piped in:

...At this point I would ask her: *What do you mean by 'just'?*

I was immediately struck by both the simplicity of the question and the profundity of it. Clearly, *just* meant more than *just* in that context, and Dr. Frankel was showing me how words can be used to obscure and hide a less than benign intent. In this regard, this woman often used what in group therapy is a group scapegoating technique called *intrusive introspection* where the person being questioned is subtly encouraged to feel doubts about his/her motives/meaning so that they become both self-conscious and isolated in the group. In this regard, it is surely not surprising that this type of *questioning* had been done to this group member in her own home, that is, done to make her doubt herself around her disturbed (Borderline/dysregulated and destructive) mother.

Summary of Chapter 3 and Implications for What Is Soon Going to Happen in This Book

Beginning with *The Psychopathology of Everyday Life* (1901) and *Jokes and Their Relation to the Unconscious* (1910), Freud extended his understanding of the unconscious mind. He did so by using the insights that he had gained from the psychoanalysis of neurotic patients. Starting with the observation that neurosis is an unconscious defense against intolerable experience, Freud now looked at a variety of normal phenomena, such as slips of the tongue, which had previously been thought to be accidental, and jokes, where he demonstrated that joke telling, like dreaming, neurotic symptoms, and *Freudian slips,* all follow an orderly process where there is a release, or a blocking (repression), of thoughts and emotion followed by a failure of the repression. However, in these phenomena, the failure of repression is temporary, and the interference with the person's functioning is minor and brief.

In parallel to these kinds of experience, during my training and my journey to become a psychologist/psychoanalyst/psychodynamic psychotherapist, I have had a number of experiences that, at the time, I did not understand, and therefore, I did not focus on them for too long, because they were quite confusing and upsetting to me. It was only later in my professional life that these experiences began to make psychological sense. I have presented several of these experiences above because the essence of my so-called magic is that I have taught myself how to *listen to a person's clinical experiences, understand, decode, make meaning of, and, finally, translate that meaning to the other*.

When a clinician becomes a Presenter, particularly when their consultant is skilled at creating an atmosphere wherein the Presenter feels both held and allowed to be *in reverie*, the result is often a heightened pull *to express and confess*. In fact, we have already seen bits of this above, and we will soon be seeing more below, in even greater detail. Further, as part of the creation of a 'holding place for reverie,' a skilled Consultant can often become quite attuned to the preconscious processes. I am describing by being continually alert to them. In a similar fashion to the skill building that occurs in the making of an experienced clinician, a skilled Consultant/Supervisor will over time develop a 'well-stocked mind' (Shulman 1982 in Mendelsohn 2022)[6] that makes the creation of a space for holding/reverie, and the facile making and testing of clinical hypotheses, a relatively straightforward endeavor.

In this chapter, I have described my use of humor, sarcasm, and phrasing when dealing with seemingly impossible clinical situations and/or when I want to make an important interpretation quickly and powerfully. I have also discussed the power of words to influence and expand (or inhibit) communication in the clinical setting.

In this regard, I presented examples of a series of words and/or phrases that convey a double meaning to the listener, and just as with the gratuitous remarks of a Presenter, I both listen to and employ such words and phrases when teaching my clinical approach. I do this to demonstrate that the use of a particular word or a phrase, at a particular time, conveys more than one meaning, and sometimes, the double meaning of the word or phrase conveys certain preconscious pulls to influence the listener.

As we have already begun to see throughout this book, our unconscious/preconscious system is very creative and is the source of important clinical information. I see my work as an extension and elaboration of all that we have talked about above, Freud's work, followed by the work of several later theorists (Reich, Reik, Winnicott, Bion, etc.) who have each helped me to more deeply understand the many unusual experiences that I have had as a clinician/supervisor and teacher of psychodynamic psychology and psychotherapy. Each of these experiences has taken me to the place where I am today, a place/approach to clinical phenomenon that many of my students and former students have called *magical,* but I have described instead as a series of processes and functions that are both teachable and learnable.

Finally, in this chapter, I have highlighted a group of phrases and processes as examples, because the spoken word when used thoughtfully in a clinical setting can be understood to have much more power than the hearer, or perhaps even the speaker, consciously knows. As we translate these processes by decoding the meaning of our patient's dreams and our Presenter's communications in later chapters, I believe that you will see more clearly how my *magic* works.

Notes

1 I am not a stranger to *strange experiences.* Prior to training as a psychologist and during my college student days, I spent time working as a drummer in several bands and for both Al Kooper and for the Rock and Roll singing group—The Ronettes. The Ronettes were a girl group from New York City, and they became one of the most popular Rock and Roll groups of the 1960s; one of the Ronettes' most famous songs (recorded after I left for my graduate studies) is "Be My Baby." At the time, like many musicians, I consumed my share of *substances.* However, the experiences that I have referred to above occurred well after (seven to ten years after) I had given up substances. By the time these events occurred, I was practiced in both thinking clearly and (I hope) acting responsibly.

2 Reik, T. (1948). *Listening with the Third Ear.* New York: Grove Press.

3 The translation of a metaphor is one way to understand and decode the hidden (preconscious) meaning of an enactment, that is, the meaning of an act or behavior out of the patient's awareness, that occurs in a therapy—typically as an attempt by the patient to work through their traumatic childhood. We have already seen many such enactments and their translations throughout this book.

4 Bernard Frankel was a veteran of World War II who survived the Battle of the Bulge and helped liberate the concentration camp at Mauthausen before going on to influence generations of group therapists. Dr. Frankel was a Clinical Professor at Adelphi University's Postgraduate Programs in Psychoanalysis, Couple Therapy, Group Therapy Training, and Supervision, where he headed the Group Therapy Training Program. He was also a former Director of the Group and Family Therapy Department at New York Roosevelt Hospital's Department of Psychiatry. As early as the 1970s, Bernie was an outspoken, direct, humorous, and smart teacher and presenter, both nationally and internationally. His beard and ponytail, impish grin, and willingness to ask uncomfortable questions made a lasting impression on all who knew him, worked with him, and learned from him. Adelphi University Day Residue 2021.

5 See note 4.

6 The screen memory contains earlier, contiguous, and later memories that serve as an important guide to dynamics that help to determine how we developed our personality in childhood. C.F., Freud, Sigmund. 1901. "The Psychopathology of Everyday Life." *The Standard Edition of the Complete Psychological Works of Sigmund Freud, Volume VI,* vii–296. Throughout this book, I will be demonstrating that the experiences that we use in decoding our unconscious reactions to a patient or supervisee can come in many forms. Sometimes, it appears as a memory of some music; sometimes, it is a powerful emotional experience; sometimes, it is a barely noticeable change in one's feeling state; and sometimes, it is a strikingly powerful image(s) like the ones that I presented above.

References

Coleman, M. (1956) Externalization of toxic introject. *The Psychoanalytic Review*, *43*, 235.

Erickson, M. (1964) 'A hypnotic technique for resistant patients: The patient, the technique and its rationale. *The American Journal of Clinical Hypnosis, VII*(1), 4–8.

Freud, S. (1901) The psychopathology of everyday life. In J. Strachey et al. (Trans.), *The Standard Edition of the Complete Psychological Works of Sigmund Freud* (pp. vii–296). London: Hogarth.

Mendelsohn, R. (2022) *Freudian Thought for the Contemporary Reader*. London: Routledge.

Nelson, M. C. (1981) The paradigmatic approach: A parallel development. *Modern Psychoanalysis, 6*(1), 9–26.

Reik, T. (1948) *Listening with the Third Ear: The Inner Experience of a Psychoanalyst.* New York: Grove Press.

Sherman, M. H. (1981) Siding with the resistance in paradigmatic psychotherapy *Modern Psychoanalysis, 6*(1), 485.

Sherman, M. (1998) Siding with the resistance in paradigmatic therapy. *Modern Psychoanalysis, 6*(1), 47–64.

Shulman, M. (1982) Intelligence and adaptation. Psychoanalytic Review, 69(3), 411–414.

Spotnitz, H. (1976) *Psychotherapy of Preoedipal Conditions.* New York: Jason Aronson.

Spotnitz, H. (2004). *Modern Psychoanalysis of the Schizophrenic Patient: Theory of the Technique.* New York: YBK Publishers, Inc.

Chapter 4

What Is Parallel Process and How Does It Enrich Our Understanding of Psychodynamic Case Formulation and the *Preconscious Transmission* of Clinical Data?

The Parallel Process

A phenomenon can occur in psychoanalytic supervision and in case formulation where a patient's conflicts, impulses, and defenses are unconsciously communicated to the therapist who then unconsciously communicates this same material to the supervisor; this phenomenon is an important dynamic in the supervisory process. In fact, it is the process that was being enacted in the parody of 'me' and a 'student/Presenter' in the Derner Skits (above). Because much of what occurs in this scenario is unconscious, it appears to be magical. In this regard, it is not different from many preconscious processes that occur within each of us.

Thus, a person might suddenly (out of nowhere) think to themselves:

...I haven't had a headache in a very long time.

Then, as if by *magic*, the person feels the beginning of a headache. What has happened in this instance is that the pain of the headache had been 'pushed' into the preconscious, but keeping it there was only a temporary measure, and when the defenses (in this case, *negation* and *denial*) failed, the person suddenly *experienced* in consciousness—what they had been experiencing preconsciously but had, until feeling the headache, been defending against it with their conscious mind.

The parallel process is also an example of this.

Bromberg (1982) suggests that the *parallel process* occurs when:

...The supervisee with no *apparent awareness* (italics mine) is behaving with the supervisor like the patient is behaving with him.

(1982, p. 110)

Like *projective identification*, there are those in the psychoanalytic community who doubt whether this *parallel process* phenomenon exists, or, if it does exist, they believe that there is no consistent, coherent psychological explanation/ principle(s) available to explain it.

For example, Baudry (1993) suggests that there are many problems with the concept of the parallel process. He believes that, like the term 'character,' the term

DOI: 10.4324/9781003375944-5

'*parallel process*' is purely descriptive and not explanatory. He states further that finding examples of *parallel process* has become something of a *fad*, particularly among beginning therapists:

> ... During my supervisory seminar, many supervisors proudly point out some phenomenon as an evidence of the parallel process and stop there as though they had explained some event. What is usually referred to is, an apparent similarity between some incident in the treatment and its seeming re-enactment with the supervisor. The facts are, unfortunately, much more complicated. The parallel process is only a vague descriptive label applied to a multitude of phenomena, only a few of which would qualify as "true" parallel processes. What is required, in addition to the surface similarity, is a dynamic and structural congruence between the two situations. This is often difficult to demonstrate, because so many 'of the crucial dynamics 'of the participants are unknown or can be inferred only with great caution.
>
> (1993, p. 610)

I agree with Baudry as to what is required to identify an experience as part of a parallel process, but I suggest that this process is a much more common one and that it is the most dramatic example of the operation of projective identification in both the supervisory and the Consultant relationship. This is because the parallel process stimulates powerful countertransference reactions that result in inducements of thought and feeling, as well as enactments of these thoughts and feelings. More to the point for our purposes, I believe that an awareness of the parallel process in all its subtleties will quickly alert the supervisor/Consultant to essential aspects of a clinical presentation *before they are consciously available to the Presenter.* As one might imagine, when this occurs, the supervisee might experience his/her teacher/supervisor/ Consultant as performing something 'strange and mysterious.'

Projective identification is a defensive operation that, I believe (2009), operates in all intimate human relationships, including the relationship that occurs between the patient/ the therapist and the supervisee/the supervisor. I also suggest that this process has a profound importance for the understanding of each kind of clinical relationship, that is, the relationship between patient/therapist/supervisor, and even between the therapist (albeit indirectly), the supervisor and the patient. However, because all of this seems so complicated, it is important to present many examples of these so-called magical processes, because as one unravels the dynamics of each case presentation, the principals involved are simple to observe/easy to teach/easy to learn.

History of the Concept of Parallel Process

Ekstein and Wallerstein (1958) provided the first full description of the *parallel process*. These authors described supervisees who seem to act in parallel with their patients, in both the supervision and the therapy. Eckstein and Wallerstein suggested that in most instances, these therapists are actuaries mirroring their patients' issues because of the similarity in dynamics and defenses between themselves and their patients.

Doehrman (1976) attempted to show that the parallel process can occur from many directions and that it can even originate in the supervisory dyad and be brought back into the therapy treatment relationship by the supervisee, as opposed to the process as it is typically described as originating in the interaction between the patient and the therapist/supervisee that is then brought into (enacted) in the supervision. Doehrman found that the therapists/supervisees she studied acted in the treatment in ways that were reflective of, or in opposition to, their perceptions of how their supervisors were behaving with them. As one example, a therapist who felt that his supervisor was authoritarian and critical would stimulate the therapist to act in those ways with his patients.

Many who have examined the *parallel process* consider that supervision and therapy each creates both dyadic and triadic relationships. Wolkenfeld (1990) and others (Billow and Mendelsohn 1982) describe the *parallel process* as a triadic one, involving the supervisor, therapist, and patient, as well as the complex interactions among them. In their understanding of the *parallel process* literature, Miller and Twomey (1999) suggest that the typical notion of the *parallel process* has presumed that the phenomenon is caused in some way by what has occurred in one dyad, linking that dyad to others, and that the link is through identification. I have suggested that this is the process that was being parodied in the Adelphi/ Derner Skit that was presented about me in the Preface at the beginning of this book (Arlow 1963; Doehrman 1976; Wolkenfeld 1990).

To summarize the above, I have suggested that while some writers question the universality, frequency, and utility of the *parallel process* concept in psychoanalytic supervision, you will soon see many examples below that demonstrate how much the supervisory and the Presenter/Consultant relationships stimulate *parallel thoughts/feelings and pressure toward enactments* in both participants, which make each member vulnerable to displaced enactments with their patients as well. Thus, the concepts of the intersubjective field and of relational dynamics (Frawley and Sarnat 2001) are found to be so important in current psychodynamic psychotherapy, and they have also been uncovered in psychoanalytic supervision, adding an important dimension to understanding the interactional dynamics of the patient, the therapist, the supervisor/Consultant. These processes have been labeled *the parallel process* in psychodynamic supervision, and I will demonstrate that understanding these *parallel inducements and parallel enactments is what a skilled clinical supervisor can learn to do in order to increase his/her understanding of the hidden meanings in the clinical encounter that would otherwise make little or no sense.*

What Is Projective Identification?

As has been described above, projective identification is a term first introduced by the child psychoanalyst Melanie Klein (1946). It refers to a psychological process in which a person strives for emotional balance by engaging in a particular kind of projection. Projective identification differs from simple projection in that it is a kind of interpersonal self-fulfilling prophesy whereby one individual relates to another in such a way that the other person alters their behavior to make the projector's belief true. However, it is understood that this induction of a self-fulfilling prophecy is unconscious rather than overt. The very nature of unconscious inducement makes this kind of communication more powerful and, if not adequately understood, potentially more malignant. As we see repeatedly in this book, projective identification is a common mode of communication between intimates, and therefore, it is not necessarily seen only in disturbed, e.g., borderline and psychotic, populations. Projective-identificatory communications are attempts on the part of each member of a dyad to influence the other, that is, to incite the other member into feeling/action states. Projective identification may be indicative of borderline and other serious psychopathology in one or both members of a dyad when it appears as a part of a complex of other primitive defenses, such as omnipotent control, but it is not necessarily pathological in every case. Traditionally, projective identification had been understood as a developmentally early and primitive psychological process and one of the more malevolent defense mechanisms (Klein 1946; Kernberg 1975; Ogden 1977). Yet, McWilliams (1994) suggests that while projective identification can still be seen as a pathological defense, ironically it can also be thought to be the psychological process out of which more mature psychological functions, such as empathy and intuition, are formed. In her book *Psychoanalytic Diagnosis* (1994), McWilliams points out that projective identification combines elements of projection (attributing one's own feelings, thoughts, and motives to others) and introjection (incorporating the feelings, motives, and thoughts of others). Thus, as has been suggested above, projective identification validates one's projections by making the projections real. There is also room in this conception of projective identification for the possibility that an individual employing the defense has seen and recognized something real—though latent and unconscious—in the other person, not merely made it come about. This recognition of the other's unconscious content is the common thread between projective identification and empathy.

Considerable empirical data, garnered particularly by Lachmann and Beebe (1996) indexing the nonverbal matching behavior of partners, indicate that partners induce similar affective and subjective states through facial expression alone. Again, although this attunement to a mate is essential to making a shared life run smoothly, it is also what makes couples and other dyads susceptible to projective identification and to confusion about boundaries and inside/outside. Grotstein (2005) sees projective identification not only as an unconscious, omnipotent, intrapsychic fantasy (i.e., as the process described by Klein 1946) but also as consisting of two other processes: (1) Conscious and/or preconscious modes of sensorimotor induction and/or evocation or prompting techniques (mental, physical, verbal, posturing or priming, 'nudging') on the part of the projecting subject, followed by (2) an interpersonal process, that is, a mode of communication between psychoanalyst and patient, not necessarily pathological.

In two previous papers (Mendelsohn 2009, 2011 and in my book *A Three Factor Model of Couple Therapy* 2017), I explored the defense of *projective identification* in couple's psychotherapy.

Projective identification (PI) is typically considered a characterologically primitive defense mechanism. As it often occurs in a muted, covert way, some clinicians view the concept with skepticism. Others view it as a process seen exclusively in very disturbed patients. I suggested that projective identification is, in fact, a common mode of communication between intimates and therefore not necessarily seen only in disturbed dyads. I also suggested that there may be other, less malignant motives involved in PI between two people. Many PI maneuvers are enacted without the conscious awareness of the parties involved, through projecting and then identifying (i.e., acting as if the projections are true). For example, when one member of a romantic couple comes home and greets his/her partner for the first time that day and senses the partner is in a bad mood, he/she might begin acting defensively, reifying their partner's original feeling. Soon, a kind of self-fulfilling prophecy has occurred, and one person's bad mood is now a looming conflict between them.

These non-verbal transmissions of fantasy, feelings, and/or action seem to fit the description of projective identification, and they can occur in many kinds of intimate human contact, including the psychodynamic dyad, as well as in the psychodynamic supervisory relationship. That is, I believe that these eliciting maneuvers can occur, from the patient to the therapist to the supervisor and back again, and that they occur through projective identification processes. Moreover, I suggest that what has been referred to as *the parallel process between supervisor and supervisee* is the operation of projective identification between all three of the following parties: the patient, the therapist, and the supervisor.

Timing Is Everything—Particularly in Psychotherapy with Couples

I had previously presented my belief that the most important process in clinical practice is the timing of the clinician's interventions, and I had placed this in broadleaf because this process suggests that one act differently when working with patients versus working with students/supervisees.

I also presented a silly joke that I tell my students about the importance of timing.

Here Is a Clinical Anecdote about a Couple

I believe that it will demonstrate not only the processes involved in *timing* but also much of what we have been talking about so far, in terms of the *preconscious transactions* that we will soon see occurring in all the parties: in this example, it can be seen in both members of the couple and their therapist (*me*):

I had been working with a young couple (I'll call them Amy and James) for several months. They were unsure about whether they were ready to move to the next level in their relationship and plan for their wedding or should take more time to decide if the relationship was right for them. Each had previously been married for a short time, and each had been through a traumatic divorce. They seemed to love each other, but they were scared.

My Office Setup

The way my office is arranged: there is a desk and chair behind me, two comfortable leather chairs that face each other and share an ottoman, and a couch that is directly to my left, or to the right of the person(s) who would be sitting in the chair opposite to me.

During one somewhat heated session, James began to express insecurity about Amy:

Whenever I come into the bedroom you quickly get off your phone.

Amy's retort also showed insecurity:

But you never let me see your texts.

I took a deep breath, waited, and let myself "feel the room." Something felt different. I now asked:

I know this might sound strange, but are you both feeling closer and more like you want to marry?

At this point, James almost shouted, "This couch is very uncomfortable!"

Then he quickly jumped up, almost bounding off the couch and into the chair opposite to me, but on the other side of the room from Amy. Shockingly, Amy continued to talk about their phones and their trouble with closeness, and soon James was also talking about this. *But nothing had been said about the literal distance that James had now put between himself and Amy.*

I waited. I waited more. I felt that if I now pointed out how James had run away from Amy and that Amy hadn't noticed, I would be putting each of them on the spot. James is a somewhat proper, uptight, but very decent man who spent his childhood caretaking a depressed mother while his somewhat inadequate but bullying father belittled him. Amy had a wonderful relationship with both parents until she entered puberty, at which point both parents seemed anxious and rejecting of her—*ran from her*—because of her budding sexuality.

I continued to wait for the right time, which arrived when Amy began to talk about how there were times that James acted uncomfortable with her in public and

James acknowledged that he was often worried that she was *too demonstrative*. As we explored these dynamics, James said to me, as if prompted:

> It's amazing how much you can read into things. I feel like you really understand us.

I saw this as permission, that is, *the right time*, to talk about how much I love the mind and how exciting it is to observe people and help them by understanding them. Now I had my chance. I talked about what had happened earlier in the session with James's changing seats and how I had waited because I knew that he had been belittled as a child, while at the same time, James's father had abdicated his responsibility to both James and James's mother. I also pointed out how wonderful it was that Amy hadn't noticed that she had continued to talk and that this allowed James to feel comfortable enough to hear this now.

There was a long silence, one of those silences that are rich with meaning and that feel like things are changing within a couple. In fact, I think of these moments as a time when both are separating from old defensive patterns—in this instance, fear and shame and avoidance of intimacy. Following this, both James and Amy talked about their love and commitment to each other, and I felt a deep sense of joy as well as a sense of relief.

As we can now see, there is certainly much to talk about in this vignette: inducements, enactments, and a projective identification–fueled transference–countertransference matrix. In the sorting process that all clinicians do, I chose to talk about none of this with this couple. However, we can see that because of all the complicated processes as well as the dynamics of the couple involved, it was particularly important to wait until my intervention could be experienced as having been done with care/protection and love.

To restate, timing is important because a sense of timing helps to make both the patient and the therapist less vulnerable to participating in enactments via inducement of transference–countertransference feelings, and more likely instead to gain understanding when such enactments occur. Further, the clinician is less likely to simply participate in an enactment without understanding it because he or she has allowed themselves the "time" to reflect on what's going on in each member of the clinical encounter. In this vignette, we can see that: *Struck While the Iron Was Cold*, so that all of us had moved out of the negative space we were in, and therefore, all members of the triad were less vulnerable, and all were thinking and feeling more clearly.

To complete this picture, I want to emphasize what I have said before: Projective identification is an unconscious identification.

I want to briefly remind us about this process via Freud (1917) who began to look at unconscious identification in psychoanalysis while he attempted to understand the mechanisms in depression.

In a depression, one is not only sad but also hating oneself and reproaching oneself and that doesn't happen in pure mourning. At first, this whole situation didn't make sense to Freud. Perhaps, Freud suggested, in mourning, there's an actual loss, but in depression, the person is reacting to a loss, but it is an *internal loss.*

Freud reconstructed the process as follows:

Person A is attached to person B. There's some disappointment; that is, Person A disappoints Person B. Their relationship is shattered. Person B emotionally falls down; however, soon they pick themselves up and dust themselves off, and move on.

However, it is not the same for Person B Prime.

Person A Prime is attached to Person B Prime. There's some disappointment, that is, Person A Prime disappoints Person B Prime. Their relationship is shattered.

Freud concluded that the melancholic/depressive is reacting to some internalized loss in the same way as the mourner is reacting to a real loss. In some breakups, one person might mourn a little and go on. But another person might go into a depression.

He reasoned: the depressed person maintains the attachment even though they can't maintain the relationship. How do they do this? They regress. Depressive people are oral. We've all observed that infants put everything in their mouth. The first relationship we have, our relationship to the world, is through the mouth. Depressed persons can't maintain the relationship, but at least they can maintain the attachment. Person B Prime emotionally swallows Person A Prime.

In this regard, you might remember the dream of the young man, the cannibal dream that I had presented above. This was a very regressed image of what the experience of the depressive process is, a primitive process like the man on the hospital ward who kneeled and made the sign of the cross (an example I have also referred to above). So, the person can't maintain the relationship, but instead maintains an attachment by identifying, that is, by swallowing the "other" who has disappointed them.

I propose that the *magic* that I have continually referred to throughout this book develops out of the clinician learning how to open oneself up to the experience of identification with his/her patients and students/supervisees. I also suggest that most clinicians already do some version of this every day in their work with their patients. However, many of them aren't aware that they are doing it! As Aron (1996) suggests, when we open our minds and allow ourselves access to the unconscious experiences in the clinical encounter, these experiences become more available, and we become more aware of clinical data that have been there in the room all along. As I have said from the beginning of this book, I believe that experienced clinicians perform *magic* but that this magic follows principles of logic, or better said, *psycho-logic,* and that the principles are both learnable and teachable.

Summary of Chapter 4

To summarize, as I've said above, employing Bion's (1977) concept of maternal 'reverie' as the capacity to sense (and make sense of) what is going on inside the infant has been an important element in our current understanding of the patient/ therapist conscious and preconscious transactions. Reverie is an act of faith in unconscious process. It is considered the equivalent of Winnicott's (1973) maternal preoccupation. In therapy, the analyst's use of 'reverie' is an important tool in his/her response to the patient's material: "It is this capacity for playing with a patient's images that Bion encouraged" (Symington & Symington 1996), and it is what I look for/gratuitous remarks/slips of the tongue/and other data in the interaction between myself (the Consultant) and the clinician (the Presenter). To have seen these processes in action, in supervision, and in case formulation is to have witnessed the power of 'reverie' to decode the preconscious transactions in the most complicated of clinical situations (Bion 1977).

As I have also suggested above, the very process of creating a *holding environment where the clinician can find a safe space for reverie* also makes the same clinician vulnerable to the patient's *projections/projective identifications and enactments,* all of which are typically not accessible to a clinician's conscious awareness. Yet, at the same time, this preconscious experience also creates a pressure for its conscious expression. When this same clinician becomes a Presenter, particularly when their consultant is skilled at creating an atmosphere wherein the Presenter feels both held and allowed to be *in reverie,* the result is often a heightened pull *to express and confess.* In fact, we have already seen bits of this above, and we will soon be seeing much more below, in even greater detail. Further, as part of the creation of a 'holding place for reverie,' a skilled Consultant can often become quite attuned to these preconscious processes by continually being alert to them. In a similar fashion to the skill building that occurs in the making of an experienced clinician, a skilled Consultant/Supervisor will over time develop a 'well-stocked mind' (Shulman 1982). This *'expanding mind'* encourages the creation of a space for holding/reverie, as well as the facile making and testing of clinical hypotheses, into a straightforward endeavor.

References

Arlow, J. A. (1963) The supervisory situation. *Journal of the American Psychoanalytic Association, 11*(3), 576–594.

Aron, L. (1996) *A Meeting of Minds: Mutuality in Psychoanalysis.* New York: Routledge.

Baudry, F. D. (1993) The personal dimension and management of the supervisory situation with a special note on the parallel process. *The Psychoanalytic Quarterly, 46,* 56–70.

Billow, R. M., & Mendelsohn, R. (1990) The interviewer's presenting problems in the initial interview. *Bulletin of the Menninger Clinic, 54*(3), 391.

Bion, W. R. (1977) C f, Personal Communication, In R. Mendelsohn (Ed.), Critical factors in short-term psychotherapy, *Bulletin of the Menninger.*

Bromberg, P. M. (1982) The supervisory process and parallel process in psychoanalysis. *Contemporary Psychoanalysis, 18*(1), 92–111.

Doehrman, M. J. G. (1976) Parallel processes in supervision and psychotherapy. *Bulletin of the Menninger Clinic, 40*(1), 4–104.

Ekstein, R., & Wallerstein, R. S. (1972) *The Teaching and Learning of Psychotherapy.*

Frawley-O'Dea, M. G., & Sarnat, J. E. (2001) *The Supervisory Relationship: A Contemporary Psychodynamic Approach.* New York: Guilford Press (Dr. Frawley O'Dea is a graduate of our doctoral program).

Freud, S. (1917) Mourning and melancholia. In *The Standard Edition of the Complete Psychological Works of Sigmund Freud, Volume XIV: On the History of the Psycho Analytic Movement, Papers on Metapsychology and Other Works.*

Grotstein, J. S. (2005) 'Projective transidentification': An extension of the concept of projective identification. *The International Journal of Psychoanalysis, 86*(4), 1051–1069.

Kernberg, O. (1975) *Borderline Conditions and Pathological Narcissism.* New York: Jason Aronson.

Klein, M. (1946) Notes on some schizoid mechanisms. *The International Journal of Psycho-Analysis, 27*, 99.

Lachmann, F. M., & Beebe, B. (1996) Chapter 7 The contribution of self- and mutual regulation to therapeutic action: A case illustration. *Progress in Self Psychology, 12*, 123–140.

McWilliams, N. (1994) *Psychoanalytic Diagnosis.* New York: Guilford Press.

Mendelsohn, R. (1978) Critical factors in short-term therapy. *Bulletin of the Menninger Clinic, 42*(2), 133–149.

Mendelsohn, R. (2009) The projective identifications of everyday life. *The Psychoanalytic Review, 96*(6), 871–894.

Mendelsohn, R. (2011) Projective identification and countertransference in borderline couples. *The Psychoanalytic Review, 98*(3), 375–399.

Mendelsohn, R. (2017) *A Three-Factor Model of Couples Therapy* Lantham, MD: Lexington Books/Rowman & Littlefield.

Miller, L., & Twomey, J. E. (1999) A parallel without a process: A relational view of a supervisory experience. *Contemporary Psychoanalysis, 35*(4), 557–580.

Ogden, T. H. (1977) *Projective Identification and Psychotherapeutic Technique.* New York: Jason Aronson, Incorporated.

Shulman, M. A. (1982) Piagetian developmental psychology. *Psychoanalytic Review, 69*(3), 411–414.

Symington, J., & Symington N. (1996) *The Clinical Thinking of Wilfred Bion.* London: Routledge, pp. 12–13.London, UK: Routledge.

Winnicott, D. W. (1973) *The Child, the Family, and the Outside World* (p. 17). London: Middlesex.

Wolkenfeld, F. (1990) The parallel process phenomenon revisited: Some additional thoughts about the supervisory process. *Psychoanalytic Approaches to Supervision, 1*, 95–109.

Chapter 5

Magical Processes in Psychotherapy and in Dream Interpretation

Let us now turn to some clinical examples of the beginnings of my so-called magical skills in psychotherapy and case formulation. From these early examples, we will see the roots and the development of my current approach, that is, my use of all the extant conscious and preconscious data to formulate and plan psychodynamic psychotherapy for myself, as well as for my student/Presenters. While this approach has been called *magical* by many, it is simply the application of several processes to each clinical case. This application exposes data that may not have been clearly available data that can enrich and make new meaning to understand each case and formulate a successful treatment plan more deeply.

Case Example 1

Early in my psychotherapy training (in the mid-1970s), a colleague and I rented an office to share. I was delighted with the arrangement; she was an excellent and like-minded professional companion; she was also quite neat, I am not. The office, while modest, looked terrific. Unfortunately, this arrangement lasted for less than a year. My officemate and her partner soon bought a house, and she built her own office into their residence. I was now left with a larger rent, and after only a few months, I am somewhat embarrassed to admit this—my office was in some disarray.

The patients I had been working with for some time either didn't seem to notice this growing mess or they felt they needed to take the good with the bad. However, a new patient (a young male attorney) came to me for a consult, and he was very upset at my office 'mess.' As he wasn't wrong about the state of the rooms, I apologized but added my own question:

> ...I apologize for the 'mess'...BTW, is there also something about this office *mess* that troubles you-- *for any other* reason?

The question sent this man into a fury, and he spent the entire rest of the meeting in righteous indignation at my *unreasonable question*. He then left, saying he was never coming back. BTW, my question came directly out of my psychoanalytic

DOI: 10.4324/9781003375944-6

training: ask questions that might move the conversation from the surface to the depth of an issue, and outrage over *mess* can be an exaggerated concern about all messes, that is, it is a common kind of concern with people who struggle with serious obsessive/compulsive issues.

I did not hear from this patient again for over a year. Then, to my surprise, he came back to see me because his closest friend, the person who had also seen me for a short period and had originally referred this man to me, urged him to come back. This time, he had a *Confession to Make*. He had, in his own words, *made a mess* of his life. First, he had gone along with a rather controlling girlfriend and gotten engaged and then married (he claimed that he had not wanted to do this but felt coerced). And while he had been thinking about leaving the law firm where he worked as an associate and starting a joint practice with a close friend and trusted colleague—his finance and his father had convinced him to stay where he was, and thus, he had turned his friend down. Now, he felt that he had also lost a wonderful opportunity with his friend who was already doing well in solo practice. In short, this man reported that he had (again) *made a mess of his life by not following his own instincts.* In this new session, the patient now went on to describe his struggles with his autocratic father who the patient described as a *know-it-all* and with his passive mother who the patient felt had been his father's accomplice and apologist. Further, he stated that, in our first meeting, when I had focused on the word *mess*, it had sent him into a state of dysregulation. At that moment, he had felt that he had to escape from me, and at the time, he had taken a page from his father's *playbook*; that is, he had become condescending and demeaning toward me, as his father had always been to him. BTW, he was correct in that this kind of background (autocratic/know-it-all parent(s)) can lead someone into having no confidence in their own decision-making abilities and also that it tends to create within the person a deep-seated rage toward those authority figures who have helped them to doubt and undermine themselves; in fact, all of these issues had actually been displayed by this man at his initial visit, but I hadn't known it.

That is, I cannot say for certain that, at the time of his initial visit, I had understood these processes in him. Perhaps, I had just, as I originally thought, focused on the word *mess* by following rules that I was learning in my training. However, the major lesson from this incident was clear; everything in a session *means something*, although at first blush one might not know what it means. BTW, remembering this incident also makes me think of the dilemma that some clinicians must have when they are training in certain behavioral techniques using required training manuals. It would be a great irony if some of the so-called science-based, empirically supported treatments using manualized techniques only work (when they do work) *by accident.*

Case Example 2

Some years later, I was treating a young woman using a modified psychoanalytic approach. The patient was a resident in a medical specialty, and she felt that she was in a very difficult life situation. Fortunately for the therapy (if not for her), I had worked with several young women in similar situations prior to this, so I was neither surprised nor unequipped to handle what was to come.

First, some background about her history: The patient had what she described as a very inadequate father and two very inadequate brothers. In the 1990s, when I was treating her, I would not have thought about the issue in this way, but I would now describe all three of these men as having been on the Asperger's spectrum. And the father seems to have had more severe Asperger's than the sons. The family lived on the West Coast and my patient had come east to college and medical school; she was now in her residency. The patient described her mother as a very 'nasty' woman who had always been very disappointed with her own husband and her sons, felt that she had married down, *and repeatedly said this to her daughter*. I don't know all the things that the mother said, but I know there were remarks made to this young woman when she was a girl that were all on the order of:

...Find somebody smart, not these schmucks...

That's not really a great thing to do to a child: if you feel it, work on it—but certainly, keep it to yourself.

While in college, this woman met a young man, who was in law student at the same ivy-league school. They fell in love, got married, and then he quickly flunked out of law school. It was unclear why. I am guessing that it is not an easy feat to be granted admission to an excellent law school and then to flunk out! What I had learned about this man's background was that his father was a ne'er do well; he called his father *a loser*. In any case, this young man now had seemingly *recovered from his upset about law school* and he had grand plans, but these plans seemed to me to be psychopathic plans involving trading stocks in a kind of *boiler room* situation.[1] While my patient was a resident in a very prestigious medical residency, her new husband seemed now to be *in training* to be *a crook*, and my patient wanted to have a baby. And, she said that she loved this man. (Perhaps one could say that she loved him because he was a loser like her dad, and/or maybe one could say that her dad was more loving than her mother had been, even though he didn't make much of his professional life.) However, can you see the difficult situation here? Because she was now saying, in each session, how things were going to *soon* must come to a head. She was about to be finished with her residency, she wanted a child, he needed to get a *real job*, she was stressed out of her mind about this, she loved him (perhaps for neurotic reasons, but she loved him nonetheless), and she didn't want to lose him, yet she might have to. As I have said, over the years that I had been practicing as a clinician, I had several cases like this before and I worried that this might not end well for my patient or for the therapy.

For several sessions, this (now anguished) young woman kept going back to how he was *not* like her father, how brilliant he was, and how talented he was.

Now, this was not a strict psychoanalysis, I no longer employed treating the person on the couch, but she came to sessions three times a week. I don't work that way now, but that's how I was trained and that is how I worked then.

In the incident that I want to talk about, at one scheduled meeting, the patient came running into my office and she was over 10 minutes late. This was very unusual. As she rushed to the couch, she said that she had: "...*I lost my way*" ...that is, after all this time coming to see me, she suddenly hadn't been able to remember how to get to my office! She sat down in her chair facing me, out of breath, all upset. I must say that this is not the first time that I had this kind of experience, in similar circumstances, and this helped me understand what I needed to do. I was now going to look for clues in my preconscious associations with what was occurring...and follow these clues to whatever place they took me.

While in reverie, the number ten (as in 10 minutes late) suddenly appeared in my mind's eye. I went with my *mind's eye 'hunch'* and I asked:

...What comes to your mind when you think about when you were 10 years old...?

Having regained her composure and having caught her breath, she replied:

... When I was 10, I overheard a fight between my mother and my father, and I suddenly realized that my mother was going to divorce my father - she called him a *loser*. They divorced later that year. But I loved him anyway. ....

To underscore what had happened here, this person was a bright, decent, mildly obsessional, and very organized person, who suddenly forgot where she was going...*as if she were a lost child who is afraid, confused, and in need of help and facing a traumatic loss.*

Following the model that we have been talking about above, I made a *connection* between this patient's '*symptomatic act*,' that is, her lateness (cf see comments above regarding Freud's *The Psychopathology of Everyday Life*, 1901)[2,3] as well as the patient's current conflict with her husband and her *childhood conflict with her parents.*

But why had this specific number appeared in my head? I believe that this woman's (unusual) lateness and her association with her upsetting childhood discovery about her father were a message to both of us that she felt that she and her love relationship were *running out of time.*

Shortly after this incident, the patient came to a session and reported that her husband had suddenly quit his own psychotherapy and she also confessed that he had been threatening to do so for a while because he believed that his therapist was critical of his vocational plans (this was something that she had not told me/perhaps she was afraid to tell me—perhaps this was a reenactment of her traumatic childhood where I had now become her critical and hateful mother—and if she told me, then I would condemn him and her).

Not long after this episode with the lateness, and her *confession* about her husband's therapy, the patient and her husband separated.

In a postscript to this story, sometime later, this patient began a relationship with another medical resident, and they later married. This woman has corresponded with me over the years to share the news of the birth of her children, the sudden death of her father, and several other milestones in her life. BTW, like several physicians that I have treated over my many years of clinical practice, particularly those in certain medical specialties where one sees lots of death, for a long time this woman would suddenly and seemingly out of nowhere contact me to ask how I was. While I never said this to her directly, I think that we both knew she was checking to see if I was still alive and well.

How can we understand the *magical question about numbers* that came to me in the session?

I believe that this young woman's out-of-character lateness was dynamically determined that she was enacting a state of regression into a bewildered, pre-adolescent child—a child who couldn't think as an adult and so could…at least for a brief moment…not let herself be aware that her relationship with her husband was nearing an end. Just as when one picks up a phone call and hears horribly upsetting news and then yells *'Oh no!'* in the first moments after the 'No' has rung in the ears—the person has bought themselves a few seconds of ignorance by way of the process of denial. In a similar fashion, this young woman *bought a few minutes of bewilderment, confusion, and the avoidance* of the painful reality that was crashing in around her.

The Magical Process of Dream Interpretation

In the history of psychoanalysis, one important example of the preconscious transmission of data occurs in the clinician's interpretation of the patient's dreams. With the realization that dreams are an expression of the unconscious, Freud (1900)[3] acquired a deep understanding of unconscious processes. Others before Freud had posited the idea of a relationship between dreams and the unconscious, even those of very early civilizations such as the Sumerians of Mesopotamia.[4] However, Freud's psychoanalysis brought a new level of understanding and new ways of working directly with the unconscious mind. While others saw dreams as meaningless occurrences, over 120 years of psychoanalytic clinical work, as well as work in sleep research and neuroscience,[5] has demonstrated that dreams are the product of both the mind *and* the brain.

The Interpretation of Dreams (1900) is often considered Freud's greatest work. It was stimulated by Freud's analysis of the dreams of his patients as well as by his self-analysis. In interpreting both his patients' and his own dreams, Freud recognized that he could apply the free association method to dreams. A dream is made up of a manifest content and a latent content. The manifest content is the dream as it appears to the dreamer upon waking and the latent content is the dream as it is unraveled after the method of psychoanalysis is applied (free association and detailed inquiry). The manifest content involves the dreamer's most recent needs, worries, and concerns (called the day residue: events of the past 24 hours have left a kind of residue of experience inside the dreamer), while the latent content concerns unconscious wishes. In presenting this model, Freud suggests that dreams are not the result of random brain activity. In this way, Freud was agreeing with the writers of antiquity who believed that dreams contain meaning. However, Freud was also suggesting that, although to the ancients the meaning of the dream comes from outside the self, to Freud the dream's meaning is psychological and comes from within. Freud also proposed that dreams have a second purpose: They preserve sleep by discharging powerful emotional experiences that have accumulated during the day. When interpreting a dream, it is essential to understand that the dream is *a lock to be opened* and that the patient's reported day residue *is the key to the lock.*

Unraveling the Dream: The Day Residue and the Process of Reconstruction

The same process that occurs in our unraveling of the preconscious meaning in each of our Presenter's *gratuitous remarks* is the process that has long been described in unraveling the meaning of the dream. That is, decoding a gratuitous remark and correlating it with the dynamics of a case is part of the same long tradition that began with the technique of free association/reconstruction/ interpretation in Freud's (1900) psychoanalysis of symptoms and dreams.

Further, as Freud (1900) demonstrated, young children display obvious dream images/symbols in their dreams. However, as each of us gets older, along with age there is a corresponding maturation of cognitive abilities, language skills, psychological defense mechanisms, and coping methods. As this occurs, we adults advance to using more and more complex verbal metaphors disguised as images in our dreams.

In sum, the same process that I have suggested is operative in the decoding of the *magical* understanding that one can observe in case presentations can be observable in the decoding of the dream.

Example:

Here is a somewhat typical example of a patient's dream in a psychoanalytic psychotherapy session and its decoding:

The day residue:

A male employee is called into his (female) boss's office for his *Annual Work Evaluation and Review.*

While the evaluation is primarily positive, he does get a few mixed evaluation comments about some minor aspects of his job performance, along with suggestions for ways to improve these. The boss presents all aspects of the Review to him in both a helpful and respectful way.

That night, he has a dream:

...I show up on a workday at the office, *but I realize that I am naked!* That's it...I feel embarrassed and humiliated. The dream ends with my attempting to find a place to hide...

After this patient's (male) psychoanalyst has asked for details about the day residue, the patient begins to associate with the dream; he remembers many times during his early adolescence when his father wanted to have a *father/son talk*—often instigated by mother when she was angry with the patient over some chore that he had forgotten or some other minor infraction. The patient further remembers that he would later overhear his father telling his mother that his father had given the boy: *a dressing down.* He then further associates to how, after a while, he began to consciously provoke his mother and purposely 'forget to do a chore' …hoping against hope that his father would tell his mother that she should *go easy* on her son because he was "…*a very good kid*… (This '*very good kid*' phrase was another term that the father would sometimes use during the patient's childhood to describe the patient, that is, the father would describe the patient this way when the patient had not angered his mother.)

As this patient associates further, he also begins to think that he may sometimes purposely *forget* certain tasks at work, perhaps to 'piss off' his (female) boss. Here the therapist adds that the patient may still be looking for his childhood father to save him and intervene on the patient's behalf, and the therapist adds that all of this is a kind of *enactment* that seems to be an important theme in this patient's life— at his work, in his therapy, and in the patient's own marriage.

Examples of the Dream Interpretation Process

Here are several other examples of dream interpretation mirroring the same processes that occur when a consultant is decoding the Presenter's *gratuitous remarks,* but in this instance the Consultant is looking for the latent content of the dream, while the equivalent to the Presenter's *gratuitous remarks* is the day residue of the patient, as reported by the Presenter:

1 The dreamer is a 30-year-old, cis-gendered man, who has recently begun psychotherapy because he is afraid to commit to marriage with his now pregnant girlfriend. The day before the dream he had accompanied her to a prenatal exam.
   The Presenter is his therapist, a 46-year-old cis-gendered man.

   …Ihadaseriesofdreamsaboutmanywomengettingpregnant-*butnotbyme*…and I kept wondering in these dreams…who's the father? How did this woman get pregnant…and there was this one dream that was very upsetting! In that one - I'm sure that I am *not* the father of all of these children, but someone says that I am the father…

At this point, the Consultant asks the Presenter about the patient's relationship with his own father.

The Presenter replies that the patient never knew his father and that he is the child of a mother and her affair with a married man.

The Consultant says the following: "I want to ask you an unusual question… does this man ever fanaticize about his biological half-siblings?"

"Yes, he does" … is the Presenter's reply.

The Consultant now says the following:

> This person's history, his dream and his presenting problem suggest a long-ing to be part of his natural father's original family and to, on the one hand, be *like* his father and, on the other hand, to have his father as the parent to him that he never had. In the therapy an important theme would be to help the patient become a *good father to himself.*

Here is another:

2   The Presenter is a 33-year-old, white, married, cis-gendered female. The patient is a 58-year-old white, cis-gendered female who had entered therapy to work on her feelings about the end of her 30-plus-year marriage. She recently reported a dream about her ex-husband:

> I dreamed that I was talking to my best friend about him, (my ex) and I told her that I thought he was special at his job- but then-all of the sudden- I said '…Oh he's just a *hack'* –but I've never used that word…

The Consultant now asks: "Do you know about the patient's history. For exam-ple, did anyone in her family of origin drive a taxicab?"

The Presenter answers: "Yes…her father. She talks about him as a ne'er-do-well both as a father and as a provider. He failed at several businesses, through-out her childhood and adolescence, and when he was desperate for money, he would drive a taxicab to pay the bills… he was always in and out of money and always moody, withdrawn, and depressed…"

The Consultant now suggests that the Presenter explore the ways the patient be-lieves that her ex-husband is like her father and the ways that she believes *that he is not similar*. The Consultant also suggests that the patient is working hard, at least in her preconscious, to protect her husband from her own contempt for him—the kind of contempt that she had while growing up for her own father who was often forced to be a *hack*; this is a slang (and often demeaning) word in America for a taxi driver.

The Presenter agrees and notes that she (the Presenter) didn't understand the historical context that was being triggered when the patient said that she worried about her children's feelings about their dad and that the patient had told the Pre-senter that she was particularly worried about her two 20-ish year-old daughters. Now, the Presenter thinks that she will begin to focus a bit on what ways the patient's ex-husband is *not like* the patient's father. She had believed that part of this patient's working through the trauma of the end of her marriage was to feel and express anger at her ex-husband. She now realizes that, while this is so, the situation is a bit more nuanced than this.

The Consultant also suggests that the Presenter (and others in the audi-ence) visit the work of Robert Langs (1976)—a psychiatrist/psychoanalyst who suggested that patients in psychoanalytic psychotherapy sometimes attempt to unconsciously *supervise* their therapist via their own associations and dreams. Here is another:

3   The Presenter is a 35-year-old white cis-gendered male. The patient is a 41-year-old cis-gendered female, married with two adolescent children (a 13-year-old boy and a 15-year-old girl). The patient reported her dream as having occurred the night of a very serious and traumatic fight with her husband:

> I dreamed that I had to have my legs amputated and I would now have to be in a wheelchair. In the dream, *I was surprised that I wasn't more upset about this.*

The Consultant now asks:

> Has the patient been struggling with serious concerns about the future of her marriage?
> The Presenter answers: "Yes, they have been having some very difficult times. She also associates that her own (the patient's) parents got divorced when the patient was 14 years old…an age that is right in the middle of her own children, (ages 13- and 15-year-old).

The Consultant comments that the dream suggests that perhaps this patient is attempting to find a way to keep herself *crippled* so she is not *mobile enough* to leave the marriage *and thus she will then be forced to stay in it.* That is, what seems to be crippled, i.e., blocked and blunted in the patient, is her thoughts and feelings about her conflictual past and the effects that this past is having in her present life.

In this regard, the Consultant now suggests that the Presenter focus questions on the patient's history and her memories centered on the trauma of the breakup of her original family. As this is discussed and looked at in depth, the Consultant reasons the patient will begin to understand whether or not *she wants to be crippled* so she won't leave her marriage and repeat her mother's past or whether *she feels crippled in her marriage* and therefore that the dream is a warning to herself that she needs to resolve herself to this failed relationship, *even though it is a repeat of her parents' (and her own) history.*

The Presenter agrees with this approach and expresses relief that things now seem a bit clearer and that she now has some new ideas about how to proceed.

Comment:

It is important to note here that, particularly in this example, the Consultant has not concluded with an *answer* to the questions raised in this presentation; instead, the presentation has led the two of them to an important area of inquiry, and it is hoped that this inquiry will make the Presenter's future work with this patient both meaningful and helpful.

As we can also see, the *key to the lock* of the dream's interpretation is the same as the *key to the lock* of the Consultant's 'magical' constructions, that is, it is a search for the preconscious links to the current problems with an emphasis on reconstruction of the present with the past. This is the same process that occurs when the Presenter and Consultant look together for clues to the patient's current dynamics by looking at the Presenter's preconscious associations to a case.

To Summarize from What Has Been Presented above

Most people dream at least four times per night (Aserinsky and Kleitman 1953) but most people remember only a small bit of each of their dreams, as the latent content of each dream is disguised via the processes of the dream- work (that is, condensation and displacement). However, occasionally a significant amount of latent content will break through the censor relatively undisguised. This typically occurs when a person is in distress and/or they have access to very primitive psychological defenses without the protection of more mature, sophisticated defenses. We have reviewed several presentations where the Consultant has understood a patient's dreams. This has enabled the Consultant to deepen the Presenter's understanding of aspects of their patient's dynamics that had previously been unclear. We will later see an example where the Consultant hears a Presenter's own dream which had occurred following a clinical encounter with his patient, and this dream will help the Consultant and the Presenter deepen their understanding of the clinical material of the case.

Notes

1 A boiler is a place where high-pressure salespeople sell, sometimes fraudulent, securities. They use the lists to identify victims of previous scams.
2 Freud, Sigmund. 1901. "The Psychopathology of Everyday Life." *The Standard Edition of the Complete Psychological Works of Sigmund Freud, VI.*
3 The translation of a metaphor is one way to understand and decode the hidden (preconscious) meaning of an enactment, that is, the meaning of an act or behavior out of the patient's awareness, that occurs in a therapy—typically as an attempt by the patient to work through their traumatic childhood. We have already seen many such enactments and their translations throughout this book.
      (See Mendelsohn, R. (2022) *Freudian Thought for the Contemporary Clinician: A Primer on Psychoanalytic Theory*. London, UK: Routledge).
4 'Dream interpretation' was prominent in early civilization (Kramer 1961). The ancient Sumerians in Mesopotamia left evidence of dream interpretation dating back to at least 3100 BCE.
5 cf Aserinsky and Kleitman (1953).

References

Aserinsky, E., & Kleitman, N. (1953) Regular occurring periods of eye motility and concomitant phenomena, during sleep. *Science, 118*(3062), 273–274.

Freud, S. (1900) The interpretation of dreams. In *The Standard Edition of the Complete Psychological Works of Sigmund Freud, Volume IV* (pp. 1–627). London: Hogarth Press.

Langs, R. (1976) *The Bipersonal Field.* New York: Jason Aronson.Mendelsohn, R. (2022) *Freudian Thought for the Contemporary Clinician: A Primer on Psychoanalytic Theory.* London: Routledge.

Chapter 6

'Magical Processes' in Case Formulation

Throughout this book, I have suggested that there are certain *truth*s in psychodynamic psychotherapy treatment, as well as in case formulation. Further, I have suggested that once a clinician understands these truths, he/she can more easily make *quick and accurate* judgments about most clinical cases.

Thus, for example, in the first interview, a clinician with at least some experience doing psychotherapy *knows*, intuits, suspects, feels and much more about their patient than they will remember in later sessions. I am not the first clinician to say this. In fact, in 1946, Alexander and French (1946) presented the following analogy:

> In the earliest (initial) interview with one's patient, the clinician can be compared to a person on a hike; the person is standing on top of a hill overlooking the countryside over which he or she will soon be traveling. At this time, it may be possible for this traveler to see the whole anticipated journey in perspective. However, once he or she has descended into the valley, their perspective needs to be retained in memory or else the image will quickly vanish. Now, down in the valley, this hiker will be able to examine small parts of the current landscape in much more detail than was possible when viewing it from a distance however, *the broad relations will no longer be so clear.*

In effect, like the experiences of a pre-verbal or barely verbal young child, all clinicians *soak up* their experiences with their patients just like a sponge soaks up water—yet, just like this barely verbal child, a clinician that is unaware of the above process will then quickly leave what he/she knows in a *space* alongside their original perspective, and often, this space is soon forgotten.

Here is a dramatic example of how I have personally forgotten important data about the initial session with my patient(s) over time:

> Many years ago-while I was in training to become a psychoanalyst, I saw a young woman for an initial consultation. She was attractive; neatly dressed and a quite composed person; at the interview, she answered my questions briefly and succinctly; she was always very clear. Given all of this, I couldn't

DOI: 10.4324/9781003375944-7

understand why I was so bored in the session. Perhaps-I thought- it was that she simply answered my questions but added nothing more to the discussion- so I was left with very little to work with. In fact, I realized after she had left that I hadn't been able to *think clearly* during our meeting. I had gotten many facts but no understanding of her current life-as if she had been filling out a written intake form with brief and lifeless sentences. In the next, follow-up session, I asked her about her childhood-while pointing out that we had only briefly touched on this. At this point the patient became quite upset; she recounted that when she was a young child her mother had had several long hospitaliza-tions for depression and that during these absences-she had been cared for by a somewhat harsh- and very controlling aunt. After this telling, the patient had then unleashed deep sobs while she also acknowledged- that -for much of her life- she had sacrificed her feelings to be good and cooperative-and- also to prevent her mother and her other caretakers from abandoning her. During this second meeting, with its very powerful exchanges, I noticed how easy it had been in our first meeting to cooperate with this patient's control in her *holding both of us at bay.*

Her initial complaint: what brought this young woman into treatment—now also made sense; close relationships always started well but ended soon after with the other person withdrawing from her. One former boyfriend had put the problem in clear focus:

> You are very nice and very sweet but there is always something missing…I just don't know if (it is that) you don't like me… or that you just hide…

The above description seemed to connect directly to her history, as she had also been told that she had been a very cooperative child. At this point in the session, I remarked: "Yes, cooperative but lifeless…"

After these two early meetings, I had made a clear determination that I would have to always be alert to this dynamic (a re-enactment) of this person's traumatic childhood and of her earliest adaptation to it.

Let me remind that reader that I was still in training, and one year later, I was in a clinical seminar where each candidate had the opportunity to present a case to the class at our weekly meeting. However, the student that had been scheduled to present their case was absent from this class. The instructor asked for a volunteer and seemingly out of nowhere (even to me), I said that I would present a young woman that I had been working with for about a year (I also noted to myself that this would be a good thing to do as I realized at that moment that I hardly ever thought about this patient except during our sessions, and for a brief moment after, when I made a few notes about her). Soon after I began, the instructor remarked that I didn't sound like my *regular self*, that is, I was droning on in a rather boring, lifeless way. Others in the class then remarked about this as well, and suddenly, in my *mind's eye*, I pictured a somewhat horrifying image: this young woman had her hands grasped around my throat and my hands were grasped around her! When I described this image in the seminar, the instructor called it a *death grip.* It was now instantly clear to me what this meant in terms of the dynamics of the case. That is, in her childhood, this woman had learned to *play dead*—in other words, she had learned that it was best to make no demands on her caretakers and to act dead and lifeless in a pathological identification with her deeply depressed mother. However, what was very surprising to me (in fact remarkable) was that I had known this in the first few interviews; I had noted it to myself, cautioned myself about it, and then *I had promptly put it out of my mind!* At first, I rationalized that I had been caught up in the details of this person's difficult life, and while that was true, it was not the point: *I had lost the perspective about her that I had had in the first few meetings, and I had lost her in the process.*

Magical Processes in Case Formulation

As suggested, I have proposed that there are always some clues to show us that a Case Presenter probably 'knows more' and often 'says more' in their presentation of a case, than he/she realizes. This process is much more common than many clinicians know. In my Consultations, I will often jokingly refer to the wonderful clues that a Presenter will mindlessly drop as *gratuitous remarks.* In this regard, in my work with both my patients and my students, I often use humor, sometimes to blunt what might otherwise sound like a harsh or critical comment from me. Thus, in this instance, when I point out a gratuitous remark or comment during a Case Presentation, I might add: "…And, BTW, you know, gratuities are supposed to be for wait staff, valets, uber/taxi drivers and etc."[1]

In what follows, I will present a number of examples of how the processes that I have described in Case Formulation often unfold between the Consultant (in this case, that is always me) and the Presenter (most typically an advanced doctoral candidate in clinical psychology, or a junior colleague or a postdoctoral candidate in psychoanalysis/psychoanalytic psychotherapy; the latter postgraduate students come from a variety of disciplines: clinical psychology/social work/psychiatry/ nursing and mental health counseling).

Examples of the 'Gratuitous Remark Process' and How One Derives Meaning from It

First, here is some background information as context for the format that I use in all my Case Consultations.

In the examples that follow, I begin each Case Consultation by asking a series (a repertoire) of demographic questions. In this regard, I always ask the same questions and I always ask them in the same order; this helps me to maintain a sense of certainty and reliability during the interviews. BTW, the questions I ask are not so different from the ones that I was taught to ask when I was trained to perform a Mental Status Interview in hospital settings, some 58 years ago, (Mendelsohn and

Harmatz 1977 and not so different from the case that I presented in my supervision with Bion in 1976 (Mendelsohn 1978)!

The questions that I ask concern the following information about each patient:

1   Age, Race, Sex and Gender Preference
2   Level of Education Achieved
3   Current Employment
4   Current Living Arrangements
5   Romantic Relationship/Status

In this regard, except under unusual circumstances (you will later see one or two examples of what I determined to be an unusual circumstance), *I do not vary the sequence of questions, and I do not ask for, nor do I want to hear, what has been listed as the patient's presenting problem(s) before I have completed my own list of questions!* In fact, most of the time I do not want to hear the patient's and/or the clinician's description of the patient's presenting problems at all, as I am hopeful that we will be able to enrich our discussion of what I might consider to be *the actual presenting issues* via the current presentation (and these presenting issues may or may not be the same issues as those perceived by the patient or the Presenter at this Case Presentation). That is, I consider a consultation most successful when I/we have been able to shift the clinician's perspective based on my approach to the consultation.

It also is important to know that I treat the Presenter's *gratuitous remarks* during the consultation in a similar way to how I might treat the *day residue* of a dream, as reported by a patient in a psychotherapy session. That is, when a patient reports the day residue that had preconsciously triggered a dream, the patient is also providing the interviewer with the key to opening a door to the latent content of the dream, just like the so-called off-hand remarks that the Presenter is offering the Consultant are an opening to his/her latent/preconscious understanding of their patient(s.)

I will return to this issue below, but for now I want to say a few words about why I ask the questions that I ask, and why I ask these questions in the sequence that I ask them:

1   Age, race, and gender preference: These questions are vital to place the patient into the major categories of intersectionality.
2   Level of education achieved: The current pandemic has put into even more sharp relief the role that level of education has in such vital life issues as healthcare and even issues concerning life expectancy. For adults, in rather stark terms: (a) less than a high school diploma, (b) a high school diploma, (c) some college credits, (d) college graduation, and (e) some graduate education are gradations that often have life or death consequences. Further, the lack of these educational advantages often points toward a severe trauma history.
3   Current employment: Related to #2, how one earns their living is a predictor of many issues regarding his/her current level of functioning in the world.

4 Current living arrangements: This information is always important under every circumstance as a clue to one's day-to-day living/functioning. That said, when one is dealing with a person who is somewhat or very disturbed, these data are often even more important. We will see how important this issue can be in several of the case examples seen below.
5 Romantic relationship/status: In an overall assessment of one's emotional health and well-being, problems in love and attachment are often a major source of emotional difficulties. Relatedly, a patient's 'love circumstances' can also be a source of resilience and strength.

The above is a very quick outline of what I ask and in what sequence I ask it. That is, "why I do, what I do, and when I do it!"
   However, it is also reasonable at this point to ask the following:

Why it is that I don't ask about- and that I actually discourage- questions/comments about the patient's presenting problems- at the very least, until we have gathered all of this preliminary data (BTW, by the point that we have established these preliminary data, I hope to have arrived at my own understanding of both the patient's actual presenting problem(s) *and* a preliminary case formulation which may be-and often is- different from the presenting problem(s) as described by the presenting clinician and the patient)!

Here is my answer to why I discourage any discussion of the presenting problem(s) before we have at least some very specific data:

As I have said throughout this book, I believe that clinicians learn about their patients in a variety of ways- and that they experience/understand each patient on both a conscious and on a preconscious level. As you have also seen, my students' (and some of my colleagues') understanding of my Case Consultation work is that it an example of a mysterious process. However, as I have said throughout this book- there is a much less glamorous explanation to my skill in case consultation- an explanation that makes it more accessible to all clinicians. It concerns the identification and presentation in the presenter of preconscious information that the presenter already possesses. Thus, I discourage the labeling of the presenting problem to not lead us astray with the patient's (and often the Presenter's) more surface understanding of the problem; so that I-and hopefully soon-we- can focus on the preconscious understanding of this case; an understanding that I believe the presenting clinician often-at some level- already knows!

That said, ironically, over the many years that I have been doing Case Consultations in this way, even with Presenters that have presented to me before, there is almost always *a powerful need in the Presenter to tell the assembled their version of the Presenting problem, a pressure to do so that is at least mildly frustrating to the Presenter.* Why is this so? I believe that there are two reasons for this and that neither of these reasons is typically consciously accessible to the presenter.

First, psychodynamic therapy is difficult, anxiety-producing work, and it makes one anxious if they begin to feel that they don't quite (consciously) understand what is occurring in the treatment of their patient. Therefore, most clinicians (even students) typically want to get the presenting problem heard and discussed because this is, at least, what the patient (and also the clinician's supervisor if they are currently a student) had agreed upon as the person's current problem, even if further exploration will show—and the clinician actually understands preconsciously that this understanding of the patient's issue(s) is not quite accurate.

Second and related to the first reason is the issue of cognitive dissonance (Festinger 1957).[2] According to this theory, when two actions or ideas are not psychologically consistent with each other, people do all in their power to change these ideas until they become consistent. Emotional and cognitive discomfort is triggered by the person's belief clashing with new information perceived, wherein one tries to find a way to resolve the contradiction and thereby reduce their discomfort. Thus, when one has been working in, and is therefore invested in, a particular way of working and with a particular presenting problem, it can be difficult to deal with the possibility that the work has been somewhat inaccurate regarding what the central issues are in the case.

Given all the above, it is often touching for me to witness a student who is quite invested in the person that they are working with and quite invested in the treatment that they are performing and then to observe this same student suddenly *pivot and change* their approach to the patient while under the weight of new/contradictory information.

Case Examples

What Follows Are Several Case Presentations Where the Consultant (Me) Works with the Presenter's Preconscious Associations to (Re-) Formulate the 'Case' That Is Being Presented:

1 The Presenter is a 36-year-old, white, cis-gendered female:

Me: What is the patient's age, race, sex, and gender preference?"
Student: "She's a 26-year-old Caucasian female--- oh, and she's cis-gendered."
Me: "How far has she gone in school?"
Student: "She graduated from college in May (this presentation is taking place in October)"
Me: "Does she work."
Student: "Not yet...she's trying to get a job but she's in an unusual field..."
Me: (This presenter seems to be adding phrases such as: "not yet...but..." with an explanation- about the patient's employment; these seem to be

attempts at *protecting/explaining* the patient- as if without these expla-
nations-what I have called *'gratuitous comments',* the listener might
become critical of-or unempathic to this patient.

I now begin to listen for two opposite, but possibly related, threads; it is perhaps the
Presenter, herself, that is critical of the patient and/or it is that the Presenter feels
that this patient is particularly emotionally vulnerable, and thus, that the patient
needs to be protected even from the feelings held by this Presenter.

As the meeting continues, I ask a few leading questions about both threads,
such as:

Do you believe that this patient is doing everything possible to find work?
   Do you ever feel that this patient is very emotionally vulnerable and in need
of protection?

What soon emerges from these questions is that in fact, the Presenter feels both reactions
mentioned above and soon the Presenter associates with her own (i.e., this Presenter's)
role in her own family of origin that she (the Presenter) was often put into the place of
a parentified child by an emotionally immature and vulnerable mother. In other words,
the Presenter was a protector of the vulnerable, but she herself did not feel protected
from her own vulnerabilities. This is not an unusual background/history of someone
who will later become a mental health clinician, and it often leads to both some ambivalence toward, and *identification with,* one's patient(s). The Consultant shares these
associations with the Presenter who says that she now understands something more
about this patient and says that she is also relieved to feel understood by the Consultant.

2 Here is similar case example:

A 32-year-old, white, cis-gendered female Presenter is asked my first four *standard*
questions:

What is the patient's age, race, sex, and preferred gender?
   …She's female. She's 29…she's almost 30…

The Presenter's answer to my query here is like that given by the Presenter above
(in example #1). In both instances, these two questions (as said above, always
the first two questions in my repertoire) resulted in the Presenter adding gratuitous comments (to remind the reader, with Presenter #1, to my query: "Does she
work…" the Presenter's response was: "…*not yet…she's trying to get a job…but
she's in an unusual field"* and for the current Presenter #2 to my query "How old is
she?" It was *"She's 29…she's almost 30…"*).

   I surmise in this circumstance, just as in the other, that the add-on comment
made by the Presenter *means something,* but I don't yet have enough of a sense of
things to draw any conclusions as to *what* that *something* might be.

I proceed to another question, the next question in my standard repertoire, that is, another question in the series of demographic questions that I ask in every Consultation that I perform:

...How far did she go in school?

Here, the Presenter answers: "She has a GED (this is a diploma that one gets when they return to high school after having dropped out; notice here that the Presenter is quite specific, that is, she does not simply say: "She is a high school graduate")."

I now have the following thoughts/hunches:

(1) That this patient has a trauma history because she didn't finish high school during her adolescence, but that she is attempting to (2) rectify the mistakes of her past by returning to school and finishing this part of her 'unfinished business,' and (3) that there must be a certain amount of resilience in the patient as she is making efforts to repair things for herself.

While I still don't fully understand what all the Presenter's *add-ons* mean, this is not unusual, and I remain confident that more data will help me to resolve the questions that are now floating around in my mind.

My next question is also a standard one ("...Does she work?" / And, if so, "...What does she do?"). This question is asked with certain hypotheses in mind. Perhaps these preliminary hypotheses will also be confirmed or they may be dis-confirmed by the Presenter's answers to these 'seemingly innocuous' demographic questions. Either way, my confidence is that I will have my own (personal) ques-tions answered, that is, the questions that I am asking myself in my own personal inner dialogue.

Here are the Presenter's answers to these questions:

Yes, she works and she's also applying to go to college...

These comments seem to confirm one of my (unspoken) hypotheses, that is, that the patient is attempting to repair the 'mistakes of her past' and that the Presenter sees her as having, at least, some resilience. It also suggests that this therapist/ Presenter is "rooting for the patient to succeed..."

The Presenter will soon confirm each of these hypotheses via even more comments to more questions, but something new will also soon emerge in the Presentation; under questioning, the Presenter, herself, will soon realize that she (the clinician) is worried that the patient may be pushing herself too quickly to repair past mistakes (this was actually alluded to with the add-on: "Yes, she works and she is also applying to college..." the 'operative' word here was 'also', as "She is *also* applying to college"). Thus, the Presenter's gratuitous comments can now be seen in another light; during the Presentation, this Presenting clinician has been attempting to reassure both 'herself,' me (the Consultant), and the other clinicians present that the patient will be able to succeed in her return to school even though the patient is also working in a full-time job (and, it soon emerges, that this patient is also raising a latency aged child as a single mother).

Thus, we can see that the Presenter's comments have been rich with meaning, not only 'meaning' that is conscious but also meaning that is preconscious, and meaning that speaks to this clinician's identification with what she believes to be a heroic but troubled young woman who is struggling and trying to juggle several difficult issues in her life, all at the same time.

The lesson here again, as we have seen before in this book, is that what might appear to the Presenter, and to the other observing student/clinicians, to be *mysterious* is a measured but quick investigation of the Presenter's preconscious (not-yet-conscious) deep and rich understanding of the important dynamics of the case.

3   Here is another case using the same procedures and technique(s):

A 29-year-old, single, white, cis-gendered female begins her case presentation by saying that the patient is a 45-year-old, white, cis-gendered male who is being seen at an outpatient clinic connected to a hospital and that the patient had recently been discharged from the same hospital where he spent ten days. The Presenter further comments that the patient had seemed rational for most of the session:

> ...For the first 44 minutes he was fine, but at the 45th minute he started sounding very strange...[3]

At this point, I have already begun to formulate an initial assessment and treatment plan based on the data (in particular-of course-the important data about the patient's hospitalization) that had just been presented, and, also from the Presenter's last comments, I now believe that this patient becomes dysregulated by the threat of loss/abandonment (as the session came closer to its end 'the 45th minute,' the patient started to become frightened of the impending *loss* of this new relationship, and this fright triggered dysregulation and confusion).

I now ask: "Who does the patient live with?"

This is not a neutral question, and *it is also out of sequence from my standard repertoire*. This is unusual for me, and my reasoning is as follows: if this patient becomes dysregulated by loss and was recently hospitalized, we should know whom he is close to/lives with. If I am (already) correct about this case (and this is still only a working hypothesis), much of the work with such a disturbed person will, at least initially, now need to center around monitoring his/her feeling states and his/her anxiety, as well as 'managing' both the patient's *and the Presenter's* level of discomfort and stress. This issue seems so important to the Presenter's understanding of the case and to how the patient should be treated, that I believe, if I am correct and I don't yet know this, that this Consultation should be immediately centered around this *'loss'* issue.

I find out that the patient lives with his sister and the sister's family (sister's husband and their two adolescent children) but that their relationship is strained because the patient can become disruptive when he becomes regressed. I next ask if this man's recent hospitalization had anything to do with a rift between his sister and sister's family, and the Presenter reports that the patient's recent breakdown happened when his extended family left the patient to go on a family trip. Soon after they left, the patient had a manic episode that led to his most recent hospitalization.

I now make some comments about what I believe to be the dynamics of the patient's current problem(s). That is, I suggest that the focus of the treatment might need to shift a bit to an investigation to determine where the patient might find a safer and more secure living arrangement, because his current situation appears to leave him (*and all of the other cast of characters in this story*) vulnerable to his continued regression due to loss/abandonment. In fact, the Presenter confirms this; the patient's family had urged him to agree to a day hospital treatment that includes a halfway house, live-in setting. I now suggest that the patient's pattern of fear of abandonment, regression-dysregulation-breakdown, is probably a life pattern for the patient, and we begin to talk about the patient's history. BTW, I have also found that people suffering from Bi-Polar I (Manic) disorder often use *methods of adaptation* like those suffering from borderline personality disorder; this complicates their symptom patterns even more.

I now have the opportunity to suggest some things that might be helpful to work on, including this patient's envy of his sister and her family's 'nice and livable-happy-life,' as well as the patient's deep regrets about the direction that his own life has taken.

Hearing all of this, the reader might now ask: Why hadn't I simply told the Presenter my initial thoughts as I had them so early in the presentation and why hadn't I quickly talked about what I thought my associations might mean for the case formulation/treatment? That is, why did I withhold my thoughts and instead ask more questions? We have already seen that I do not suffer from false modesty, so why did I wait?[4]

My answer is honest, and it might surprise you to hear that it is also humble. I don't ever know, for sure (i.e., I am never absolutely certain) about what I am actually going to hear in these interchanges. Thus, without confirmatory data about my hypothesis, *confirmatory data that can only come via the answers to my continuing questions*, I would be hesitant to send the Presenter astray, (i.e., to have him/her traveling down the wrong path). Therefore, until I had more confirmatory data, that is, data that lent support to my observations, I continued to ask more questions. When I was satisfied that we now had enough data to begin to formulate an understanding and a plan, I began to present my thoughts about the case.[5]

4   And another case:

The Presenter is a 32-year-old, black, single, cis-gendered female.
   I ask my first four standard questions:

What is the patient's age, race, sex and preferred gender?
Presenter: "She's a 29-year-old, Caucasian, cis Gendered female…"

The Presenter's answers to my query here are like that given by other presenters, but I note that the Presenter's answers seem a bit awkward to me. I now ask my next question: "What is her level of education?" The Presenter's response alerts me to the probability that the Presenter's awkwardness was real but that it was probably the result of the Presenter's preconscious identification with the patient. This is her reply:

…She graduated from XX College…

This is a local school, and we are both familiar with it. Yet, I didn't ask *where* this patient went to school. This seems to me to be more data that the Presenter feels/ or wants to feel a certain familiarity to the patient. I make the decision that I will now listen closely for anything that suggests a pull for familiarity/closeness in the patient/Presenter mix.

As the questions continue, first, I hear nothing else to suggest what I had been looking for until I get to the patient's current living circumstances. The Presenter now reports that the patient has moved back to her childhood home, where the therapist adds that the patient and her older sister, both adopted shortly after their births, had grown up:

… In an apartment building down the block from the clinic…

This again seems to be some confirmation of the idea that the Presenter is in a kind of *identification with the patient*, and I now suspect that this is the result of a process described as *twinning* (i.e., the Presenter is attempting to find and stay connected to the patient *as if they had shared a womb prior to birth*). In other words, it is my conjecture that there has been a process of *twinning* that has been occurring throughout the interview (twinning is not uncommon when one is treating a person who had been adopted and it is also not unusual for the adopted person to pull for/ induce/enact this process in their therapist).[6]

I now shift my questioning to the patient's history. The patient was adopted at approximately five weeks old. The Presenter also states that the patient describes a very difficult family home where conflict is frequent between her controlling and somewhat critical mother and that her father is somewhat aloof, but not critical. In this regard, the patient states that her two sisters have always been the only source of encouragement, love, and support in her family. She further states that the patient's mother can be particularly unkind to the patient. The patient describes her mother as rigid, controlling, and critical, and while both the patient's sisters are very organized in their work and school life, the patient is not, and she is often somewhat chaotic and impulsive. I also note to myself that the *Presenter* herself is contained and organized, but thankfully appears to be a very kind and supportive person.

I now say to the Presenter that I want her permission to ask her an odd question; here, the entire class laughs, because what is unsaid is that many of my questions seem at first to be very odd.

"Of course," replies the Presenter.

I now ask the Presenter if she has ever had the thought that there are some important similarities between she and her patient. The Presenter's reply is that while on the surface they seem so different, that is, the Presenter is both cis-gendered and a POC, and that both she and the patient come from very different childhood backgrounds—in fact, the Presenter has often had the sense that they have similarities, *but she can't figure out what they are...*

I now suggest that sometimes a person who has been adopted in very early childhood is looking for either a twin or 'looking for' their natural parent(s) or both. The Presenter now reveals that since she began seeing this patient she has wondered about the patient's natural mother and father and had, several times during the sessions, found herself fantasizing about the natural parents. The Presenter *confesses* that she had not revealed this in the current Presentation (or in her own clinical supervision) because she thought that it was 'weird'...*particularly because of the obvious racial difference between the patient and her.* She also says that she is now reassured that this can be part of the therapy process.

Later in the presentation, the Presenter agrees to try a suggestion that I have now made; that is, in future sessions, if/when the therapist suddenly feels a certain special connection to the patient, in fact, or feels such a *connection* in *reverie*, she will ask the patient about *how the patient was feeling about the therapist at that moment.*

In a postscript to this Presentation, two weeks later, the Presenter reports that she had asked this question about the patient's relationship to the Presenter—at the moment that she (the clinician) had drifted into *a reverie of closeness* and that this had opened up a flood of feelings and memories in the patient, about early longings to find her *real mother* as well as the patient's deep hurt that the mother who has raised her doesn't seem to like her.

Clearly, this is a valuable material, and it bespeaks to how *the adoptive mother and the patient* have continually missed opportunities for connection and instead that they have had many ruptures between them. As a Consultant, I can only make suggestions and point to avenues of inquiry that may have been missed. That said, in this instance, I am hopeful that I have helped this clinician/the other students and if I can be so immodest, perhaps even this clinician's supervisor, to broaden their perspective(s) on this case.

5 And another:

The Presenter is a 39-year-old, Caucasian, heterosexual, married male with two children and he is treating a couple.

The couple is a white, cis-gendered heterosexual couple in their early fifties; each has a child from a previous marriage; both children live outside of the couple's home.

The Presenter now answers, before being asked, the age and gender preference of each member of the couple and then says without being prompted:

> You know…the man (of this couple) is a *liar*…but I don't want to *rat him out*… so I should stop and wait for your questions…

Here the *gratuitous remark(s)* is obvious but what is its' deeper meaning? I am struck not only by the Presenter's comments but also by his *timing*; that is, he rushes through my first demographic questions before I can ask them, and he seems pressured to tell me that the husband of this couple needs a special kind of understanding and empathy, even while also suggesting that the man is somewhat morally compromised. My mind flashes to the following joke that I tell my doctoral and postdoctoral students as they are in training to become psychodynamic psychotherapists:

Timing:

When I teach psychodynamic psychotherapy to my doctoral and post-doctoral students, they often ask me to talk about the most important component of psychotherapy technique. My answer is to have one student role-play the parody of a scripted *interview* with me, but the "interview" is the setup for a silly joke.

The Joke:

The student is to say to me, "I understand that you are the world's worst comedian."
And I will reply.
Then, the student is to ask me, "What is the secret of your success?"
And I will reply again.
Here is the joke as I tell/*perform* it:

Student:	"…I understand that you are the world's worst comedian?"
Me:	"…That is correct…. I am the world's worst comedian…"
Student:	"…What is----—"
Me:	"…*Timing!*" (I say this word *before* the question is completed)

Clearly, in this example, my *timing* is totally off and that is the point I have made with my joke. One secret of success in all psychotherapy is *timing*. What is the issue with *timing* here in this Presenter's remarks?

In this example, the Presenter's rush to clarify that he wants to protect the male member of this couple, *while at the same time, he is condemning him by implying that he is morally compromised,* suggests an enactment.[7]

That is, my next question(s) will center on the possibility that the Presenter's rush to tell me is an enactment and I am beginning to think that the conflict has been both enacted in the therapy and is now also being enacted in this Presentation.

Consultant: "Do you think that this man undermines himself?"

Presenter:	"Yes, he lies about the most harmless/irrelevant things constantly getting himself 'in trouble' with his partner."
Consultant:	"Does he have anything to feel guilty about in his history?"
Presenter:	"Actually...yes!" His first wife died of cancer after many years of suffering. This man had left that marriage during his wife's illness and his child was raised in large part by his ex-in-laws. After the ex-wife died, the child continued to live with the maternal grand-parents. He now has a good relationship with his son, but this took a very long time."
Consultant:	"So, can it be said that whatever else occurs in this man's current relationship, he continues to punish himself for things that he did in his past?"
Presenter:	"Yes, I think that this is right."

What can be seen here is that the Presenter is enacting one member of this couple's *confession,* as well as enacting the man's seeking punishment in his current life, for mistakes that he made in the past (See Reik 1959 and above). While, at some level, this Presenter had understood this process, the Presenter's *gratuitous comment* at the start of the Presentation was a clue to both the power and the pervasiveness of the patient's unconscious guilt, as well as the patient's unconscious desire for atone-ment. Thus, what is being seen is an enactment of both processes in the therapy.

6 A brief anecdote that illustrates the techniques presented above:

I once delivered a short paper (at 11:00 am) during an, all day, annual conference of a professional society, where I was the featured speaker for a weekend of events focusing on this new approach to Case Consultation. When I had finished the for-mal presentation of the paper, I asked the assembled if anyone wanted to present a short excerpt of a case related to the topic, the use of preconscious metaphor in understanding one's patient.

At this point, an attendee in the audience (a young, Caucasian, woman of about 30 years of age) stood up, raised her hand, and said: *"I can present a case...pardon me (*she now yawned and smiled)*...it will help wake me up...I don't know...I woke up filled with energy...I heard you speak yesterday... but I suddenly feel very tired. "*

I now asked: "...Is the patient (to be presented) depressed?"
"Why yes, how did you know?" said the Presenter.

(How *did* I know? In fact, I *didn't* know for certain, but I did have a hypothesis, one that I had promptly tested by way of my question):

I hypothesized that the Presenter's comments suggested the following:

...I heard you talk yesterday-you can read minds-I am struggling with a very depressed person- who is enacting her depression and hopelessness in the ther-apy...I can't quite *tell you how* I understand this case, but I can *show you* how she wants *me* to *wake her from her depression.* In other words- I need to *show you* what she induces in me, so that you can *wake me up from what she does to me*--so that I can help her...

Below are nine more case presentations that follow the same format:

7   The Presenter is a 38-year-old, white, single, cis-gendered female.

I ask: "What is the patient's age and sex":
She replies:
              "...He's a 30-year-old, cis-gendered male, who reports that he is hav-
              ing problems in his two-year relationship with his girlfriend..."

I now ask if he is also having problems with the Therapist/Presenter.
    (I understand that this question is out of the sequence that I typically employ, but I am struck by this Presenter's almost urgent need to quickly/immediately tell me the patient's Presenting Problem *even though I had clearly stated in my introduction to the Consultation that the Presenter should withhold the Presenting Problem until I asked for it!*)

              "Yes, and we've been working together for four months, once a
              week, and he tells me, in every session, that I'm not helping him..."
I now ask: "Was his mother rejecting of him?"
She answers: "Yes...he reports that the mother was very cold to him- and to
              his older brother..."

I surmise that the Presenter, who presents as a very kind and supportive young woman, is feeling 'stung' by the accusation that she is unhelpful, e.g., that she is *cold and unloving.* I believe that her reaction to both these *accusations* is an unconscious *confession* (cf Reik 1959) as well as a *built-in defense:*

    ...This is a man---who has trouble with everybody--- so *it's not my fault if he is having trouble with me.*

In fact, in this enactment, (Levenson 2005) I'm assuming that the Presenter *is* worried that it's her 'fault' and therefore the protestation that '*he* is the trouble' is an attempt to reassure 'herself.'
    We explore these dynamics, and the Presenter expresses some relief and states that she feels better equipped to deal with her own feelings about this patient and the therapy.

8   And another case

A 28-year-old, Caucasian, cis-gendered male student has agreed to present a therapy case in a clinical case conference that includes the presenter, five other students, and me. I ask about the age, race, sex, and gender: preference of the patient and the student says:

"He's a young Caucasian, male; he's 29."

I then ask a few (more pointed) questions, followed by:

Consultant: "Do you think that this person is developmentally delayed---perhaps on the (autism) spectrum?"

Presenter: "I didn't think of that, but yeah, I think that he may actually be on the spectrum."

This student/presenter is also in his late 1920s; that is, he's 28 years old. Thus, to me, the first part of the sentence: "He's young" is a meaningful, but gratuitous remark. What does it mean? As I have said above, I don't know but I now have a hypothesis.[8]

9   And another

The Presenter is a 28-year-old black, cis-gendered, single, female.

Consultant: "…What is the age, race, sex, and gender preference of the patient?"

Presenter: "…The patient is a 23-year-old, Caucasian, cis-gendered, married female…"

Consultant: "What is her level of education?

Presenter: "The patient is completing her BA degree."

Consultant: "…Who does the patient live with?"

Presenter: "…She is currently living with her husband…"

Consultant: "…Do you think that the marriage is stable?"

The Presenter replies that she believes that the marriage is a happy one.

I then ask if the patient is under any emotional pressure and apropos of this question, the Presenter replies that the patient has few friends (and that she was traumatized in her early childhood by a speech impediment and severe social anxiety). The Presenter elaborates further that the patient's husband is *her only friend.* I now ask if the Presenter is worried that the patient is putting too much pressure on her husband (and on the marriage).

The Presenter replies:

…I didn't think of that, but her husband had initially wanted to have a large family. However, the patient says that the husband has recently seemed more reticent about having children…

I suggest that perhaps the husband is starting to feel that he is already 'saddled with a child' and that the Presenter may be more worried about the patient's marital relationship than she had realized. The Presenter agrees that this is possible and now associates that she couldn't quite understand why she had wanted to present this case; she believed that it was going well and that the patient was effectively working through her traumatic experiences of childhood, but the Presenter now realizes that she (the Presenter) is probably more concerned about the issue of this patient's marriage and its possible tenuous nature.

I now remind the Presenter of two things that occurred: when I asked about age, race, sex, and gender preference of the patient, she answered by adding that the patient was married, but I hadn't yet asked about this. Also, the Presenter had an unusual answer to the following question:

"Who does the patient live with?"

Here was her reply:

…She is *currently* living with her husband…

This is an awkward phrase that suggests that the living arrangement is in transition, and I was struck by it; this answer, along with the Presenter's urgency to tell me of the patient's marital status had caused me to wonder if the patient's marital relationship has become tense, awkward, and even *tenuous.*

10 And another case that highlights important demographic variables:

The Presenter is a 48-year-old Caucasian married female.
I ask about age, race, sex, and gender preference:

…He is a 23-year-old, cis-gendered, Haitian American male-born in Haiti; he came here at age 18.

Education and employment:

…He graduated in May 2020 with a bachelor's degree in finance, from XYZ University and he recently secured part-time employment as an assistant for a XX company.

Where does he live?
With his family, that consists of his parents and a 28-year-old half-sister.
What about his romantic relationships:

…He is currently in a casual relationship with a female friend, however, he initially reported to be single and first identified as bisexual…

Solely considering his age and gender, I remind the Presenter that the patient is contending with a variety of transitions—namely, his transitions into adulthood,

gender identity, more serious romantic relationships, and establishing a professional career path. By adding a consideration of his racial and ethnic identity,
as well as his recent immigration history, one can see how these may have also
impacted the patient's conscious identity issues, as well as his unconscious identity
issues. Haiti splits its culture and physical space with a seemingly disparate but
related neighboring nation. Haiti is currently in a state of chaos, so it is understand-
able why the patient's family would want to immigrate. I remind the Presenter that
she had mentioned this person's recent arrival in the US before being asked, and I
now ask the Presenter to think about the following question(s):

> ...How much of his immigration history/relatively recent arrival, troubled place
> of origin, its history, and the familial immigration history are related to this
> young man's anxieties in his life? Certainly, there exists some degree of inter-
> generational transmission of trauma that impacts his psyche, but how has this
> inherited-as well as recent- trauma affected him? And, to what degree-does it
> still need to be explored?
>
> Longevity, access to medical care, quality of healthcare, access to and quality
> of a nutritious diet, among other life outcomes- are all predicted from education
> level. Fortunately, this person's prognosis is more positive since he has just
> graduated from college. I also remind the Presenter that when I was asked about
> his employment, she responded, that: "Now, yes, he works part-time."

I suggest that this response might communicate a sense of relief as well as at least
some expressions of worry: (a) Does the Presenter feel that she (the Presenter)
is 'in this patient's corner? And (b) Does the Presenter worry about whether the
patient will do well for himself as time goes by?

The Presenter now expresses relief that she feels a certain sense of clarity and a
deeper understanding of the patient based on the cultural factors alone, factors that
she had thought about in the early interviews with this person but had not fully felt
the implications of until this presentation. She also now remembers that when she
first met with the patient, the Presenter, herself, thought about her own grandpar-
ents and about their arrival in the United States having left their home in eastern
Europe. I praise the therapist/Presenter for her openness and tell her, and the assembled students, that it is just these kinds of experiences that tell us so much about
our patients—things that we initially think of and know—but then soon forget as
the sessions continue and we become *bogged down* in the many details of the case.

11 And another case:

> The Presenter is a 35-year-old Caucasian, married female.
> I ask for the patient's age, race, sex, and gender preference:
> This man is a 40-year-old, white, cis-gendered male who states that:
>
> ...He wants to: "eliminate-his neurotic dependency'...

I now ask about his education and employment:

> The Presenter answers that the patient has had some college but did not graduate and that until recently he has had a spotty work history. He has only *recently* (the Presenter uses this word) obtained a job as a 'clerical worker' in a civil service position that has regular pay, benefits, and job security.

I now ask if the patient had begun this job after the therapy started and the Presenter says 'Yes'—that this is so.

Next, I ask about this man's romantic relationships: he is divorced; with no children. He has a girlfriend, and they live together with her two adolescent children from her previous marriage.

I now ask the Presenter to think about her opening phrase about the patient:

> ...He wants to totally eliminate his neurotic dependency'...

She says that when she now says it 'out loud,' it sounds like one might be knocking down an old, abandoned, eyesore of a building.

I agree, and I now suggest that the patient is not consciously aware about what it means to be neurotically dependent, but that it sounds like he is, in fact, *co-dependent*. In other words, it appears that this man believes that while he is emotionally involved with other people (i.e., his girlfriend, perhaps both his parents and perhaps his ex-wife), he feels that they *do not understand* him. Therefore, I suggest, the patient is effectively saying that he is: '*on strike!*' What I mean by this is that this man is symbolically holding up a picket sign and declaring himself angry and that, at some level, he feels that his neurotic traits are not '*eliminate-able.*' In other words, the meaning of my "On Strike" metaphor is that perhaps this patient is much more angrily entrenched in his dependency than even he realizes. That is, it is as if he is waiting for a message from someone who will save him from his suffering as he 'pickets against' all those who have wronged him throughout his life. I further add that from the Presenter's use of this opening phrase, it seems like this patient is locked into a kind of self-torture and demonstrates a kind of refusal to move, i.e., a kind of impenetrable 'stuck-ness.'

The Presenter now adds (in a kind of confirmation of what I have just said) that the patient and his ex-wife have been 'feuding' over their marital assets since the end of their marriage almost four years ago.

I now suggest that this man's angry dependency may be partly the reason that, until recently, he has had a spotty work history and was not able to complete college, and, further, that starting the therapy might have helped him get a more sustainable employment. Finally, I suggest that if in the exploration of these dynamics with the patient, the patient begins to feel some access to anger, what should then occur is a kind of emotional freedom and the Presenter/therapist might want to then further explore the reasons that this man *does not want to 'totally eliminate' his emotional dependency*, even though he consciously believes that he does want to do so. Finally, I suggest that the reason that he may not want to do this may be that perhaps there is something (or some things) that keeps him trapped in this emotional dependency and, therefore, trapped in his own hostilely dependent -intransigence and anger.

The Presenter now asks with some excitement:

"...So, if I understand you correctly, I might be able to say:
"Underneath all this helpless stuff, you're enraged at your family; you take it out on yourself- and then- you don't move."

I praise and applaud the Presenter for her ability to translate my ideas into her own helpful comments and language. What I don't say is that the Presenter's desire to create her *own language* is probably also an enactment in response to her wanting to 'free herself' from her patient's oppressive language about his *'totally eliminating his neurotic dependency,'* that is, it is also an enactment.

12 And another:

The Presenter is a 31-year-old, white, cis-gendered male.

I ask: "...What is the patient's age, race, gender, and sexual preference? ":
The Presenter answers:
"...The patient is a 20-year-old, cis-gendered, white female-college student living at a local college. She is struggling with a long-term (since high school) turbulent relationship with a boyfriend, and she is also having conflicts with her roommate... and she misses her mother.

I note that I did not ask for this extra information, but since I have it, I now ask about both patient's parents:

Consultant: "You said that she misses her 'mother'. Was she living with the mother? Is there a father in her life?"
Presenter: "...The mother and father have been separated for many years- from the time she was a young child (!) But- they are not divorced. The father is a successful businessman. The mother seems very disturbed and doesn't work. Throughout the patient's life, she has spent the school year with her mother and the summer and some weekends with her father. She now lives with her mother but has a decent relationship with her father. The mother appears to be very defensive, manipulative, and scheming and takes no responsibility for any of her own actions; she also does lots of blaming the external world, particularly blaming the father..."
Consultant-   "...Let me stop you here for a second... I suggest that the most effective treatment approach would be to first work with this young

woman about how *'stuck she is' and how this is related to her family situation.* That is, I would explore how her parents' inability to get a divorce is *the model* for how this whole family *'lives in the world'.* That is, there is no resolution of anything…time stands still…life stands still…. In this regard, I think that it is wonderful that this young woman lives at her college. I would also be working with her on an exploration of the family history, beyond both parents. That is, exploring the ways in which these parents can talk about their own mother and father's marriages and how all of this history might have affected *them.* In other words, I suggest that there may be a link in all of this to an intergenerational transmission of trauma. This may provide you (the Presenter) and the patient with a chance to 'fix this.'

I next say the following to the Presenter and the assembled: "…BTW, by now each of you knows a bit of how I think…weird, yes? In this regard, I wonder *who this young woman is to each of her own parents?* That is, symbolically, is she *her father's father?* Is she *her mother's father?* What I am suggesting is that one needs to look at all the metaphors. I think that what happens in this kind of case is that everyone gets so enmeshed that even the Presenter can become 'trapped' in a timeless/ever-spinning loop and that this is probably starting to happen to all of you!"

Presenter: "Yes, I see that I was feeling an urgency to tell you everything quickly or else…"

Consultant;   "…Yes! Or else *what?* I would contend that the 'or else' was that you might get trapped in the same timeless void that this family is in; this is exactly what *an enactment* feels like and I'm so glad that you are now experiencing it *and describing it in words* instead of just getting totally pulled into it…"

13 And another case to demonstrate this process:

The Presenter is a 41-year-old, white, cis-gendered female.

Consultant: "…What is the patient's age, race, sex, and gender preference?"
Presenter: "The patient is a 35-year-old, white, Cis-Gendered male."
Consultant: "What is his education? "
Presenter: "…He graduated from a Southern Bible College with a B.A…"

I note here that the Presenter has made a *gratuitous comment:* 'Southern Bible College,' and this suggests several connotations. One possibility is that ordinarily, this patient would be less likely to be coming to talk therapy, that is, if he was still very observant. Thus, it is more likely that he is 'in rebellion' from his strict religious background, and therefore, he might be estranged from his family, and that he is probably struggling with issues of personal autonomy, regret, and loss of his earliest identification objects. Of course, these are just *best guesses* based on the barest bits of demographic data (and what the Presenter felt pulled to tell/*confess* to us) but these associations can show the reader the way that I am now processing these data from the very beginning of this presentation.

Consultant: Does he have any contact with his family?
Presenter: "No, and he is depressed about it."

At this point, the Consultant quickly moves the Presenter into a discussion of the patient's fears that he must choose between his own '*authentic self*' or give up his core values to be able to reconnect with his family. Several possibilities are discussed, and the Presenter is relieved that she now understands that the issues here are about the patient's attempts to resolve issues connected to his identity and deepest (unconscious) identifications. It is suggested that the Presenter return to an in-depth discussion of the patient's (and his parents') earliest history, that is, to look for early objects of identification to help this patient understand his history more deeply.

In a postscript to this meeting, several meetings later, the Presenter discusses, with excitement, that her probing about this man's early history had uncovered the early loss (*estrangement) of his mother's oldest brother,* who had become estranged from her family of origin after he had been drafted into military service, when her mother was herself a young girl. While this information raises many further questions about this case, it does offer both the patient and the Presenter/Therapist more data to continue to help this patient make meaning out of his life and out of his current identification/autonomy struggles and also make meaning out of his current life choices. That is, it offers up that, as one possibility, this man has been 'living out' (enacting via an unconscious identification) a trauma that occurred in the very early life of his mother.

14 And another:

The Presenter is a 40-year-old, white, married female and the Patient is a 20-year-old, white, cis-gendered, single, male.
During my series of questions, the following has been established:

The patient is a sophomore in a local college, living in the college's dormitory and the Presenter points out that the college is affiliated with a Roman Catholic order and that this is consistent with some of the patient's issues; that is, the patient suffers from severe obsessive-compulsive traits-including a behavior pattern known to occur in the followers of many different religions; it is called *scrupulosity* (Miller 2008)[4]-a rigid and unforgiving concern about being a good parishioner-praying frequently, and, it seems-often berating himself for not living up to high and rigid religious and moral standards. Thus, it becomes clear that this patient's religion-like many aspects of this man's life-is being used to torture and punish his 'self.' It is also noted by the Consultant that much of what the Presenter is adding to the conversation is offered before being asked, so one might surmise that the Presenter is anxious and eager to quickly *tell the patient's entire story'*. That said, all the information about the patient is delivered in a somewhat dry, almost affectless way-even the description of the patient's major symptoms. The patient's history is described as his having been a victim of a sadistic and brutal father and a mother- who-while not physically abusive-was not supportive of him and was often verbally critical of the patient-particularly because she-too-is quite religious. In this regard, the patient reports that he always seemed to *fall short* of his mother's high religious standards and her high expectations of him. In sum, the Presenter suggests that the patient is often dissociative, very self-punishing, help -rejecting, hopeless and self-attacking. He has no romantic interests and no friends.

The Presenter now cites an example of this man's self-defeating/self-punishing style. The patient had reported an incident that recently occurred; that is, recently a strange man on the street had walked too close to the patient (this occurred during the period of safe social distancing during the Corona Virus Pandemic) and the patient had then wondered to himself:

What is *wrong with me* that the man did this?

Several other examples of the patient's self-attacking style are also presented again without affect or emotional expression by the Presenter. The Presenter then sums up what she has said with a final comment; she reports that the patient ends each session by saying the following:

Do you see that understanding things doesn't help?

I (the Consultant) now say:

So, I am some crappy Consultant…and you are some crappy therapist…even the man on the street is better than we are…

The Presenter lets out a laugh (showing emotion for the first time).
 I follow-up the above comment with the following:

So, what I would do with this patient would be to listen for *more* criticism about the you (the clinician) and then point this criticism out (I often use humor in my work-as I did just now, but there are many ways to do this- depending on one's personal style and preference). Following this, I would praise the patient for being able to *trust me enough to insult me.* That is, one might consider a strategy of *attacking the attacking parts* of a self- punisher and then reward the patient for attacking outward…especially if the outward attack is at the therapist. I now also point out that until my sarcastic comments this Presenter had been talking in a monotone voice. The Presenter now remarks-with some surprise and embarrassment, that this is what the patient sounds like. I quickly reassure her that it is wonderful that she was able to 'put herself so deeply into this patient's place' and I add that this is often what occurs with a severely traumatized person who induces (pulls for) enactments in their therapist. I further say that this is often a key to the case- and that for the Presenter-this key was *buried under the rubble of the patient's self-punishing enactments.* Finally, I point out the irony that the only person the patient can express anger towards (besides himself) is the therapist; with everyone else-even a stranger on the street-he is too frightened. While this had eluded the therapist; now her curiosity is aroused. Finally, I comment to the Presenter (and to the assembled) that when a therapist is put into (*induced into*) an enactment, one temporarily loses his/her reasoning powers- and therefore one's curiosity. Thus, one of the helpful aspects of presenting material in this setting is that the Presenter can now actually hear them-selves out loud and become self-reflective about how he/she may have been (unknowingly) participating in an enactment.

15 And another:

The Presenter is a 29-year-old Caucasian, single, cis-gendered female, and I ask:

What is the patient's age, race, sex, and preferred gender?

She replies:

She's a 20-year-old Caucasian, cis-gendered, gay female.

I then ask about education and work history and the Presenter informs us that the patient is a college student and that she also works part time.

As the questions continue, and I ask about where the patient is living, the Presenter replies that the patient lives with her mother and that her father had died of a heart attack five years before and that her younger sister had died ten months ago of a drug overdose. Then, the Presenter mentions that the mother often talks about the patient's dead sister (and sometimes about the father) as if both were still alive. I ask the Presenter for an example of this, and the Presenter says that a few times a week the mother might make a meal and remark that:

"XXX" (the deceased sister) 'really loves this…"

Or the mother might be watching a program on TV and yell out "…XX (deceased sister) should be watching this!"

I now suggest to the Presenter that she refocus her questions/comments to the patient. In this regard, the Presenter had been working with the patient on the patient's feelings of sadness and loss about the deceased sister and also about what feelings and memories this loss has triggered in the patient about her late father. I suggest that, along with this, the Presenter now focuses some of her questions and comments to questions about the patient's mother, about the mother's history/

the mother's parents/ the mother's school and work history and even about the mother's life before she married the patient's father, as well as questions about the mother's current interests (and whether the mother has any friends).

The Presenter now remarks that she knows almost nothing about both parents except that the father had died and that the patient now has two remaining older sisters (each in the late 1920s). Then, the Presenter adds: "Oh…and…both sisters live together out of the parental home…"

The Presenter now asks for my rationale about the suggested change in focus, and I say that in some families, the entire family colludes in hiding a *secret* from themselves and from each other and often from the world. I continue that in this case, I believe that the secret may be that this patient's mother is quite disturbed and that the mother seems intent on treating the children as if they (the patient and her sisters) are the *'identified patient(s)'* (that is, the *'ill ones'*). I also suggest that the Presenter's new set of questions may help the patient to begin to realize how much she may have been hiding this information about her mother from herself. The Presenter now remarks that perhaps that is why the patient's older sisters have been urging the patient to move into the apartment that these sisters share.

Postscript: At the following Case Presentation meeting (three weeks later), the Presenter asks to give an update about the most recent sessions with this patient.

The Presenter reports that as she began to ask her patient more questions about the mother, and as the patient then began to answer more and more questions, the patient also became very anxious. Further, in the two most recent sessions, the patient had now remembered that throughout her own childhood, she intuitively 'knew' that she could get no reassurance or sense of protection/safety from her mother and that she always sought out her sisters, instead. The patient further stated that she had recently made the decision to ask her sisters if she can live with them. The Presenter also reports in the session that followed this, the session where the patient had decided to ask her sisters if she can live with them, that the sisters had agreed to the patient moving in with them, and that the patient had then told her mother about her plans to move out, but that the mother had simply replied: *'Oh…'* and then the mother had walked away to her own room!

I (The Consultant) now praise the Presenter for her courage and flexibility, and I also talk about how in some family systems, the entire family's *'code of conduct'* is centered on protecting a disturbed family member (often this is one of the parents) from an acknowledgment of his/her severe psychopathology.

16 And another

The Presenter is a 37-year-old, white, married, cis-gendered male, and I ask:

What is the patient's age, race, sex, and preferred gender?

He replies:

She's a 33-year-old heterosexual female.

I then ask about education and employment and the answers are that the patient graduated with an MBA in business administration from a local college and that she is working at a start-up financial company.

As we move along with the questions, the Presenter's answers are interesting but unremarkable, until he discusses the history of the therapy:

> The patient started the therapy exactly one year ago today-in late February…

I remark that it is not February, *but October,* and the Presenter seems embarrassed, quickly apologizes, and changes his answer to the correct date.

I now ask what comes to mind about *February* (versus October) and the Presenter describes February as "the coldest month of the year…"

He then quickly adds that he is beginning to feel a certain 'coldness' from this woman that he didn't feel up until now and he adds that he realizes that *this* is the reason that he had decided to present this case to me. He also wonders if she is beginning to get ready to quit the therapy, although there has been no direct evidence of that.

I now ask if either/or both of the patient's parents had ever given this patient *the cold shoulder,* and the Presenter reports that in fact, this has always been an important metaphor in this patient's family history; that is, while the patient's father was more emotionally available and more affectionate than the mother, this father might suddenly turn on the patient; or he might suddenly turn on either of her two sisters (i.e., he is described as having had a bad temper/mean streak *and that he could suddenly turn cold on one of his children for what seemed like a minor offense and sometimes for a long period of time).*

We now begin to work on the idea of an *enactment* as a process that occurs when one is working with a person with a trauma history and the Presenter begins to feel more secure in being able to understand consciously, what it now seems he had been struggling with preconsciously (and thus, what he had presented preconsciously to us in this Consultation). I also reassure the Presenter that it is not unusual for processes like the possible enactment to lie dormant until the patient has developed a deeper level of trust for the therapist so that this enactment may be a sign of progress in the therapy. The Presenter leaves the meeting with a new level of understanding and with some reassurance about where the treatment is probably going to go next, that is, a recognition that the therapy now seems headed to a more open discussion about the role of the father's temper and coldness in this patient's history.

Comments

What I have suggested throughout this book, and what we have now also seen in these brief clinical vignettes, is that each Presenter has felt compelled to *confess* (Reik 1948, 1959) about some aspect of their Case to the Consultant and to the assembled. That is, each Presenter has often indirectly expressed a confession that has typically been about something that has yet to be explored directly in the therapy. Often, this aspect of the Case is key to some important trauma, and it has led to an inducement of countertransference thoughts and feelings via the process of an enactment. It should also be repeated that in almost every instance in these vignettes, the Consultant asks a question (or several questions) before coming to a *quick but preliminary* hypothesis and that the Consultant is willing to abandon one avenue of inquiry for another if data from the question(s) points to a different, more probable hypothesis.

I also want to acknowledge again the work of Edgar Levenson who first presented us with a deep understanding of the processes of mutual enactment. These processes are key to the decoding of clinical material in each of these cases. To quote the relational psychoanalyst, Donnel Stern:

> It seems to me that Levenson's contribution to relational thinking, via the sea change of our understanding of the nature of interaction, has been seminal, even originary; but I also believe that this influence has never been adequately recognized and appreciated by many relational writers. It was Levenson who first understood that continuous mutual unconscious influence necessarily implies mutual enactment. Does this seem to credit him too much? I don't think so. In 1972, the date of The Fallacy of Understanding, and for years thereafter, there was simply nothing else available on the subject.

Donnel B. Stern, from the Introduction - *The Fallacy of Understanding* and *The Anatomy of Change* (2005) London, U.K.: Routledge

17 And here are another two cases to illustrate these processes

The Presenter is a 31-year-old Caucasian, single, cis-gendered female.

Consultant: What is the patient's age, race, sex, and gender preference?
Presenter: The patient is a 29-year-old Asian-American female, born in Southeast Asia, and she came to the United States at age 7. She is married.

(I note here that the Presenter has offered me much more than I had asked for, particularly about the patient's early life. While this information is quite valuable and I assume that it is very important to understanding the case, I had not asked for either where the patient was born or about any of the circumstances of her childhood.)

Consultant: What is her education?
Presenter: She has a BA degree in psychology and works at a Crisis Center for Female Victims of Domestic Violence.

(Again, there is a kind of urgency to the Presenter's answers, the words seem to *pour out of* the Presenter and she is answering questions that I have not yet asked. I am struck by this, particularly as this Presenter has been a member of this clinical seminar for several months and has presented to me before. Despite the urgency that I hear, I proceed to my next question in the series. However, I already have a few hypotheses about this case, based on this current interaction.)

Consultant: With whom does the patient live.
Presenter: She lives with her husband and her mother and father.

(I note that this is the first time the Presenter's answers are neither urgent nor rushed and the answer is exactly what I had asked about!)

Consultant: In the sessions, does the patient seem overwhelmed by feelings?
Presenter: (sighs) Yes, I have trouble containing her. I don't know why her life seems to be going well.
Consultant: Is it possible that both the patient's living arrangements and her job are triggers for her distress.
Presenter: I didn't think of that-she came to therapy to talk about her ambivalence about having children. But maybe so she works with women that are in awful life circumstances. These are mostly battered women with young children. An aunt in India raised the patient, (her parents had left her to come to the US when she was two years old). She was reunited with her parents in the United States when she was seven years old.
Consultant: I now point out to the Presenter that she seemed anxious almost triggered in her initial presentation of this patient, until she mentioned the patient's husband and parents. I suggest that this may be related to an enactment where the patient is *demonstrating- via- enactment* what her early childhood was like- *until she was reunited with her parents*. I also suggest that perhaps the combination of her current work and her early life experience are acting to trigger feelings and memories that this patient is finding it difficult to consciously tolerate and/or express. In this regard, I suggest that the thought of having a child might have intensified these feelings in her. And finally, I suggest that the therapy is an opportunity to work on all of this before the patient embarks on motherhood.

The Presenter seems relieved and agrees with my assessment.

In a Postscript a few meetings later, the Presenter reports that she had suggested some of the above insights to the patient and that the patient immediately seemed less agitated. The patient also stated that until these insights, she couldn't understand her hesitancy to become a mother, and she had also felt that she was *"...letting my husband and my parents down..."* However, now the patient understands that she needs to first grieve some of her own lost childhood before she can think about bringing a child of her own into the world.

18 And another:

The Presenter is a 34-year-old, Caucasian, cis-gendered, male and the Patient is a 32-year-old, Caucasian, cis-gendered male. When I ask about the level of education, the Presenter says that the patient has a CPA in Accounting and then quickly adds that the patient has been:

…Sober for several years, and works in Finance…

These comments quickly shift me away from my next standard questions: ("Who does the patient live with?" And "…Does he have a romantic interest?"). In this regard, the Presenter will later answer both of those questions (The Patient lives with a girlfriend for several years).
    I now ask about the Patient's sobriety:

The Presenter reports that the Patient attends Alcoholic Anonymous meetings 'religiously' but that the Presenter is sometimes worried that the therapy, itself, might upset him and 'drive him into a relapse.'

I now ask if this is the reason that the Presenter had wanted to present this case, and he concurs. I next ask if there is a history of trauma in the patient's childhood, and the Presenter said that *the patient's parents had lost a child in a car accident before the patient was born.* I next ask for whatever details of the tragedy the Presenter has been told by the Patient. The Patient had reported that the child was a boy aged nine and that the patient's father had 'lost control' of the family car and crashed into another car and that *the only fatality had been the patient's sibling, a child that this patient never met.* I now remind the Presenter that he stated that he has been worrying about how he is "*driving the therapy*" and that he had expressed in this current presentation that he fears he might "*drive his patient back to drinking.*" Thus, I suggest, this presentation seems to be about an enactment of a family trauma that needs to be spoken about in words, but has not yet been fully verbalized. I now muse to the seminar about the fairy tale: *Sleeping Beauty*, and I suggest that the storyline of this fairy tale is modeled after being frozen to death; a deep sleep that mirrors the reactions that occur when a mother goes into a postpartum depression or when a fetus dies during delivery or when a young child dies; that is, when there's been a very tragic death in a family, the actual death of a child or a mother or the psychological death of a postpartum depression. I now add that when a patient comes to a therapist and the patient remembers this story as a prominent memory or a prominent theme of their childhood, the story has appealed to them because they, and their family of origin have become, in some ways, frozen in time, unable to grieve or mourn their loss. In this regard, I now reason that this patient had been using alcohol to stay *frozen* and, at some level, the Presenter has understood this. I also refer the Seminar to the recent Disney movies *Frozen I* (2013) and *Frozen II* (2019).

This leads me to a broader discussion of the concept of a *replacement child.* That is, I suggest that the current patient was *the replacement* for the parents' lost son, and I also say a bit more about the fiction in the fairy tale *Sleeping Beauty,* as well as these recent Disney full-length animated stories *Frozen I and Frozen II*[9] that I had mentioned before.

Next, I suggest that this current Presentation has been influenced by an enactment whereby the Presenter is frightened that any of his own 'careless and reckless behavior,' *recklessly driving the therapy,* will harm his patient in the same way that the patient's father was (presumed) reckless and fatally harmed the patient's sibling. This is particularly important because to help this patient to deal with, heal and master his childhood traumas, the therapy must in fact go more deeply into this patient's past, not only the past that the patient *lived through* but also in a way like the children of Holocaust survivors, to the past that occurred before this patient was actually born! The Presenter seems moved by this notion and expresses that he is relieved that his over-concern about his patient's fragility is, at least in part, the result of an enactment.

Comment: I am hopeful that it is clear in this example that the Consultant had no preconceived notion(s) about where this case was going to go but that I continued to correlate the *Presenter's* current concerns (worry of possible recklessness on the part of the Presenter) with the Patient's history (of a trauma possibly caused by parental recklessness) and the Patient's stated presenting problem (maintaining sobriety). Then, I correlated all the above with the Patient's childhood (and his current use of alcohol to blunt/*freeze* traumatic feelings, thoughts, and memories).

19 Here we see the merger of a Presenter's dream and its interpretation with a case
   formulation:

The Presenter is a 28-year-old, Caucasian, cis-gendered, male. It should be noted that the Presenter has presented material to me once before.

I ask:

"…What is the age, race, sex, and gender preference of the patient?":

The Presenter replies: "The patient is a 19-year-old, white, cis-gendered male, college freshmen."

(I note that the Presenter has told me more than I asked and wonder to myself if this is because he has presented to me previously *and/or* for some other reason).

Consultant: "Who does he live with?"
Presenter: "He lives in a college dorm, even though his family home is close by."

Consultant:	(I now believe that there is a certain urgency to the Presenter's comments, and I step out of my routine; that is, my regular line of questioning).
I now ask:	"Are you worried about this patient?"
Presenter:	"No, but I had a dream last night and when I woke up, I thought of him. I remember only a *sliver* of it..."
Consultant:	"What do you remember?"
Presenter:	"I didn't realize that it was connected but I saw him yesterday. His parents are both attorneys; he's depressed because his parents are going through a divorce...the dream was that I was looking for my car and I couldn't find it...I looked everywhere...like I said, I thought of him when I woke up and remembered the dream"
Consultant:	(I now ask a series of questions about the patient and the therapist's relationship to the patient. I am concerned about the Presenter's anxiety and whether it is related to a current worry about this patient or a chronic traumatic enactment from the patient that is being induced in the therapist but is *not necessarily about an emergency in this patient*. In this regard, it is not unusual when a clinician associates his/her own dream with their patient, but my concern was about this Presenter's worry. At this point, my questions center around the following: whether the Presenter believes that the patient has problems with his judgment; when not depressed does the patient have problems with impulse control or evidence of impulse problems/acting out; and does the Presenter believe that the patient is currently a danger to himself or others. I am relieved by the Presenter's answers to each of these questions.)
I now ask the following:	"Was this patient bullied by either of his parents?"
Presenter:	"Yes, by his mother."
Consultant:	"Was the father of any help with this?"
Presenter:	"No, and we have been working on this."
Consultant:	"I believe that you are on the right track with him. I would also suggest that you question whether this patient-himself- worries about *you*; that is, you wonder: does he worry about *whether you are 'strong enough'* to deal with the inner fury triggered by a rich and deep discussion of his childhood. In other words, I am suggesting that you are concerned that the *patient* worries about whether *you* can handle the hate growing inside of himself..."

The Presenter looks visibly relieved and remembers having a 'weird' thought during yesterday's session with his patient: *"How can I be a good father to this kid...?"*

In my (Consultant's) remarks that follow, I leave out any reference to the word 'kid,' although I believe that the word is related to the *Presenter's* worries that he, the Presenter, is also a 'lost kid' (i.e., when dealing with the patient's current enactment, the Presenter *identifies with* the patient as a 'lost kid' as seen in the dream metaphor of the *'lost car'* in the Presenter's dream). In other words, it seems that this patient pulls for the Presenter to feel helpless and impotent, as this patient believed his father was helpless and impotent, and therefore unable to protect the patient from his childhood mother. Working with this dynamic, I stress the issue of enactment, and how a patient in an enactment pulls the therapist into various regressive ego states. Related to this theme, I suggest that the patient's depression is partly connected to the patient's childhood trauma and that interpretations of the patient's aggression will give the patient permission to feel the anger inside of him-anger that this patient has probably "...fled from for much of his life...."

(The Presenter is clearly visibly relieved by all my comments).

Postscript:

> At the next meeting of this clinical seminar, the Presenter says that in the following two sessions with this patient, there was a breakthrough; the patient both expressed anger for the first time; and there was some lifting of the patient's depression. Also, the patient expressed some concern/worry, hoping that the therapy not end, until "I (the Presenter) can fix this."

These later sessions that followed the original Presentation suggest that instead of enacting his worry onto his therapist, the patient is now beginning to 'own it' as part of himself. I continue to be very encouraging and supportive of the Presenter and reassure him that he is *'up to the challenge'* with this Patient.

20 Here is a different kind of clinical situation with a complication that occurs infrequently but is important enough to be described:

All the above examples are concerned with Case Consultations where the Presenter is, at least, consciously open and cooperative in his/her presentation. What about a circumstance where the Presenter is somewhat resistant to presenting a fair, objective, and accurate presentation to the Consultant?

Healing Ruptures in the Presenter/Consultant Relationship: How to Turn a *'Presenter Enactment'* into a *'Teachable Moment'*

There is an extensive literature on the efficacy of psychodynamic psychotherapy, particularly about the process of healing the so-called splits or ruptures in the psychodynamic psychotherapy relationship (Barber et al. 2013). In fact, the healing of 'ruptures' is now considered a key component to the success of psychodynamic therapy. However, while there is some discussion of 'ruptures' in clinical supervision, (cf Frawley-O'Dea 1997) little is written about the occurrence of the healing of 'ruptures' in the Case Presentation relationship.

What can a consultant do if there is a 'rupture' (or the potential for a rupture) between the Consultant and a Clinician/ Presenter during a clinical presentation? Can such a 'rupture' be healed? Can any good from such an experience?

To further complicate matters, I will soon describe a situation that has, only rarely, happened to me during a clinical Presentation, but it is no less distressing no matter how few the 'occurrences.' That is, there are occasions where the Consultant begins to suspect that the Presenter is consciously (willfully) hiding what the Presenter believes to be some potentially damning information from the assembled about the patient/the therapist and/or about their relationship during the presentation. Why does this happen? And, further, what about when the Consultant also worries that directly confronting the Presenter about this suspicion might lead to a rupture in this public setting?

As is the situation when one performs a clinical interview with a patient suffering from 'borderline personality disorder' (Kernberg et al. 1989) in a Case Consultation interview where one suspects that the Presenter is not being totally (consciously) truthful, the Consultant often begins to suspect that what is being heard is just like in a clinical interview with a Borderline patient, 'a lot of nothing,' from the Presenter.

To dramatize what I am describing, first let me present an example of a typical 'lot of nothing interview' with a traumatized borderline patient and their clinician/ interviewer. Following this, I will present the similarities that one experiences in this kind of situation with a Consultant and a Presenter:

The clinician asks the borderline patient about their history, and what one hears is, as I have said, a lot of nothing:

"What was your childhood like?"
"A normal childhood."
"How would you describe your mother?"
"Oh, just a mother, I guess."
"And your father?"
"Just a father ... he was mean..."
Here, the clinician will be thinking:
"...We're missing data. This person is using avoidance and denial, and maybe splitting- *and I am hearing lots of nothing*" (Mendelsohn 2022)[10]

As I have suggested, while this circumstance is quite unusual, *it does sometimes also* occur in a Clinical Case Consultation/Presentation. What can the Consultant do in such an unusual and difficult circumstance?

A Lot of Nothing in a Clinical Presentation

When a consultant begins to suspect that what is occurring in a clinical presentation is a *conscious* distorting of the material (as opposed to a preconscious distorting that is the result of an inducement/enactment) *I might ask the Presenter if their patient typically gets embarrassed, ashamed and/or humiliated from revealing unflattering issues in the therapy.* This is not a neutral question (i.e., I am now in search of a kind of *pairing/parallel* of the Presenter's dynamics with the dynamics of the Patient).[11]

In fact, when I have done this, sometimes the Consultant (and assembled clinicians) will hear a dramatic 'confession' by the Presenter! That is, the Presenter will say that he or she finds 'himself' or 'herself' doing the same thing in the current meeting. In this instance, it is also important to say something helpful and like what one might do in the clinical case; it is best to now praise the Presenter, that is, to model the techniques used in dealing with a rupture in a therapy and apply those same techniques to the current Presenter/Consultant relationship.

It is also important to then say that, when such ruptures do happen, the ruptures often occur when both the Presenter *and their patient* have a history of similar kinds of trauma *as well as* a history that includes the overuse of the psychological defenses of splitting and pairing (Bion 1961, 1967).

Summary and Clarification of Chapter 6

To summarize, and clarify my somewhat unique way of formulating all clinical data in case formulation, here are the concepts that we have discussed so far in their functional relationship to each other.

I propose that in all clinical encounters, the following processes occur:

1 Along with the conscious processing of thoughts, feelings, and actions, there is an inducement of preconscious thoughts, feelings, and actions (in this scenario, most typically any pressure to *action* occurs in a kind of *inducement* process called an *enactment*).
2 All these inducements and enactments produce transference and countertransference reactions in each of the parties (patient(s), therapist/presenter and supervisor/teacher/consultant).
3 These transference/countertransference reactions are the result of both identification and projective identification.
4 All reactions in both parties in the teacher/student relationship (therapist/ Presenter and teacher/observer/Consultant) that are typically labeled as countertransference can be understood to also be examples of parallel processes because each of the parties is *inducing reactions in the other.*

Following the steps described above, in their functional relationship to each other, will allow any clinician to decode the preconscious transactions that are occurring.

Once these preconscious messages are decoded, these same messages can be used to reconstruct, at the deepest levels of meaning, everything that is occurring in the clinical encounter. This is my so-called magic that I have referred to throughout this book, nothing less/nothing more.

That said, I understand that for some readers, the above terms are both new and difficult and that my methods are at best unusual.[12] In this regard, over the years I have received many questions about my approach and also about how it differs from other Case Presentation formats. In this regard, here is a recent interchange between one of my current doctoral students and me that I suggest highlights the differences in my approach when compared to the typical format used in Case Formulation. I hope that this interchange also helps to highlight what I attempt to achieve with my own methods.

Interchange with a Student Who Had Questions about My Approach

Student: "…The process you used in class today to conceptualize XX's case was inductive: you started with small amounts of information to build a concept of what is happening with that individual. In other case conferences I've taken part in, we usually use a more deductive process, whereas the entire case is represented (large amounts of information) and then a hypothesis is built based upon the evidence presented. So my question is: why choose an inductive method rather than one that is deductive?"

Dr. M.:   "…I was not only interested in the 'facts' reported- by the Patient- to the Presenter. If I had only wanted this, I could have listened to an audio...or even better I could have viewed a video transcript of those 'facts'.

In my case formulation classes, I use a standard inquiry of the so-called facts presented by the Patient and reported by the Presenter. I continually point out that I never have a totally clear or accurate understanding of what the Patient's comments actually mean (nor of what the Presenter's comments actually mean) …BTW, I don't think that the Presenter does, either. In this regard, in the case we discussed in the class today, for me the *facts* also included the added word, 'XXX' that was part of a gratuitous comment made by the Presenter during the Presentation. As we saw when the data unfolded, this 'gratuitous word' was loaded with meaning and nuance not previously understood by the Presenter before today's Presentation.

However, I believe that this Presenter's comments displayed a beginning recognition that he understood more than he consciously 'knew' about his patient. That is, a Presenter's remarks typically alert me to the psychological fact that his/her comments mean something more than the factual, i.e., his or her conscious, understanding about the following:

1 This Presenter's feeling/thinking,
2 the patient to be presented,
3 their mix/relationship, and
4 the very act of this Presenter presenting this person to this group at this period.

The process of unraveling the psychological meaning of all of this and of putting the meaning in the context of a valuable learning experience (a learning experience that includes: (a) a viable psychological theory of motivation and etiology, (b) a technique, (c) a theory of technique, and (d) the formulation of a preliminary treatment plan for the case) is what I have begun to teach you today. I did so by describing a theory of clinical communication that includes both the manifest and latent content of patient/therapist and teacher/presenter interactions.

You will soon see why I think that no matter what a Presenter says…he/she will add meaning(s) that they are not consciously aware of during their presentation…

Student: "…Thank you for clarifying! It of course makes sense to me that the 'facts' presented are not 'objective', and that the way they are presented orients you toward the 'biases' of the Presenter. I look forward to learning further about this technique of 'finding the latent content' of both the patient and the Presenter."[13]

Summary of This Interchange

As one can see from the above interchange, the student's questions are thoughtful and move us to the heart of this clinical enterprise. BTW, what I neglected to add in the above interchange is that it was helpful that this student used quotation marks for both the words 'facts' and 'biases' as these quotation marks underscore that both the 'facts' and the 'biases' of every presentation are a matter of both the manifest and latent dynamics of the case and the conscious and preconscious 'biases' (attitudes/thoughts/feelings and reactions) of the Patient and of the Presenter. I understand that all of this adds a new level of complexity to Case Formulation. In this regard, I also want to reassure the reader that once these terms and methods are used a few times and then mastered, the rest is simply about listening closely for the appearance of these functions and correlating them to each other. Thus, what I am offering today is not so different from the way that Freud *reconstructed* a patient's history from his/her symptoms/conflicts and not so different from how he *constructed meaning* from the day residue and associations of his patient's dreams.[14]

Finally, what did not occur in this interchange is that in about one-third of the presentations that I hear from students, the procedures that I have described help us to observe new dynamic issues not available prior to the presentation. For the rest, these new procedures typically enrich the understanding of what had previously been described. I do not know why this so, but I can speculate that in this other one-third of the cases, there is a history of more severe trauma, and therefore, these patients are stimulating more inducement/more enactment in the therapist/supervisor dyad and that this may have clouded the issues in the case.[15]

Notes

1   I call the extra comments made by the Presenter as 'gratuitous remarks.' Right after I say this, I add that the comments (just like with a *gratuity*) are actually 'small gifts.' This is my real point; in this setting, these comments *are* gifts that one can use to 'decode' the presenter's preconscious transactions, thus allowing information about the transaction to then emerge; *that is why I wait for the presenter to continue before I intervene and either ask more questions or make a comment. The preconscious transactions always emerge... even when the presenter doesn't want them to emerge-as we have seen above with the Presenter who was hiding certain thoughts and feelings from the Consultant and the class.*

2   Cognitive dissonance is the perception of contradictory information. Relevant items of information include a person's actions, feelings, ideas, beliefs, values, and other things in the environment. Cognitive dissonance is typically experienced as psychological stress when one participates in an action that goes against one or more of these factors. According to this theory, when two actions or ideas are not psychologically consistent with each other, people do all in their power to change them until they become consistent. The discomfort is triggered by the person's belief clashing with new information perceived, wherein they try to find a way to resolve the contradiction to reduce their discomfort. In *A Theory of Cognitive Dissonance* (1957), Leon Festinger proposed that human beings strive for internal psychological consistency to function mentally in their world. A person who experiences internal inconsistency tends to become psychologically uncomfortable and is motivated to reduce cognitive dissonance. They tend to make changes to justify the stressful behavior, either by adding new parts to the cognition causing the psychological dissonance (rationalization) or by avoiding circumstances and contradictory information likely to increase the magnitude of the cognitive dissonance (confirmation bias). Coping with the nuances of contradictory ideas or experiences is mentally stressful. It requires energy and effort to sit with those seemingly opposite things that all seem true. Festinger argued that some people would inevitably resolve the dissonance by blindly believing whatever they wanted to believe.

3   The translation of a metaphor ("...for 44 minutes he was fine...but the in the 45th minute...") is one important way to understand and decode the hidden meaning of an enactment; that is of an act or behavior that occurs in a therapy typically as an attempt to work through a person's traumatic childhood. In this case, the metaphor was about how the patient could no longer 'hold it together' as time began to run out in the session. This was a metaphorical way to communicate to all of us that the presenter actually knew much more about the confusing behavior on the part of the patient than this presenter consciously understood. As we have seen in so many of these examples, they are each metaphor for the process of enactment in the therapy, and the translations of each of these enactments usually lead us to the major way that a patient has been attempting to master a major childhood trauma in his/her adult life.

4   Scrupulosity is characterized by pathological guilt/anxiety about moral or religious issues. It is more commonly known as religious anxiety. It is personally distressing, dysfunctional, and often accompanied by significant impairment in social functioning (Miller 2008).

5   The process that I am describing here is simply an extension and elaboration of Freud's (1912) technique of listening to the patient's free associations about the content in the patient's narrative and then asking questions in an effort to make things clearer. Freud's work was followed by the theoretical and technical advances of Reich, Reik, and others, each of which looked at the preconscious transactions that occur between patient and clinician. My contribution has been to apply these same understandings to case consultation and case formulation by translating the preconscious transactions of the presenter to the consultant and the assembled clinicians.

6 Pairing/twinning: Bion's (1961) observations about the role of group process in Group Psychotherapy have been adapted and applied to the understanding of many kinds of behavior. One concept that Bion employs in 'group dynamics' is that of the *imaginary twin*-a kind of unconscious pairing with another (Bion 1967). I have found this 'pairing' to be a common process of unconscious identification that clinicians sometimes develop with a patient whose dynamics and history has some similarity to theirs. Relatedly, patients (and therapists) that had been adopted soon after birth-or-as very young children (that is, way before one might develop a clear and accurate experience or memory of the adoption) as well as people who actually are one sibling of a pair of twins- are also prone to pairing/twinning. In one clinical experience some years ago I intuited that a patient that was twinning had been either a twin or had been adopted. In an odd twist, she was neither, but she had been born as part of a pair of twins, and while she had survived, her brother had been stillborn. This suggests that much of the issue about being a twin occurs via the parents communicating these issues preconsciously to the child and then the child *works through the twining process throughout life.* However, there are a number of other reasons that may also have contributed to this Presenter's twinning with this patient; I believe that these can be best understood via the principle of *overdetermination 6* and this suggests the power of this *twinning* process even when members of the dyad are of a different *race* and different in other ways as well. As one works with preconscious issues of diverse patients, you will begin to find that the person's issues might not *only be* about what we consider to be the most common issues of diversity; race, sex, and gender orientation (although the issues are always at least in some ways related to the dynamics) but that these issues may also be about preference for one parent over another and/ or character differences between the parents, birth order of the patient, and some other things that we might not understand from the demographic data: such as *what was occurring in the life of each of this person's parents-and in their relationship-when he or she was conceived* and/or *what was happening to the parents when he or she was born* and also *when he or she was a young child and adolescent and a young adult.* And, of course, there *is* the most obvious issue, *race.* Unfortunately, in American culture, *whiteness* is often valued over *blackness.* The psychologists Drs. Kenneth and Mamie Clark highlighted this in their research on *internalized racism,* using concepts derived from psychoanalysis and original work on projection and on *unconscious identification.* In fact, the Clark data was used in the landmark Supreme Court decision overturning the use of *separate but equal laws* employed to maintain segregated school systems. Kenneth and Mamie Clark (1958) were African American psychologists who as a team conducted research among children and were also quite active in the civil rights movement. The Clarks were known for their 1940s experiments using dolls to study children's attitudes about race, and they testified as expert witnesses in one of five cases combined into Brown vs. Board of Education (1954). Their studies found contrasts among African-American children attending segregated schools in Washington, D. C. versus those attending integrated schools in New York. The doll experiment involved a child being presented with two dolls. Both of these dolls were completely identical except for the skin and hair color. One doll was white with yellow hair, while the other was brown with black hair. The child was then asked questions inquiring as to which one is the doll they would play with, which one is the nice doll, which one looks bad, which one has the nicer color, etc. The experiment showed a clear preference for the white doll among all children in the study. One of the conclusions from the study is that a Negro child by the age of five is aware that to be "colored in... American society is a mark of inferior status." This study was titled, "Emotional Factors in Racial Identification and Preference in Negro Children," and was not created with public policy or the Supreme Court in mind, lending credibility to its objectiveness. These findings exposed internalized racism in African-American children- self-hatred that was more acute among children attending segregated schools. The research also

paved the way for an increase in psychological research into areas of self-esteem and self-concept. This use of the understanding of unconscious identification stems directly from Freud and other psychoanalysts in their work on the identification processes in the formation of the self.

7 The translation of a metaphor is one way to understand and decode the hidden meaning of an enactment, that is, of an act or behavior that occurs in a therapy typically as an attempt to work through a person's traumatic childhood. We will see many of these enactments and their translations throughout this book.

8 See Chapter 3 Parallel Process/Inducement/Enactment.

9 *Frozen* is an American computer-animated musical fantasy film produced by Walt Disney and released by Walt Disney Pictures. It's inspired by Hans Christian Andersen's 1844 fairy tale *The Snow Queen* (2002). It tells the story of a fearless princess who sets off on a journey alongside a rugged iceman, his loyal reindeer and a naive snowman to find her estranged sister, whose icy powers have inadvertently trapped their kingdom in eternal winter and whose parents had mysteriously disappeared (perished) years before. *Frozen II*, set three years after the events of the first film, follows them as they embark on a journey beyond their kingdom (Arendelle). They want to discover the origin of the sister's magical powers and save their kingdom after a mysterious voice calls out to this sister.

10 'A lot of nothing' suggests the overuse in the patient of more primitive defenses such as denial, avoidance, projection, and splitting. The result of all these defenses is that the patient is unable to report a coherent story because he/she 'can't think straight'. This is often because the patient is unable-unwilling to face very powerful, and very unpleasant, thoughts and feelings that can potentially dysregulate the self (cf Kernberg (1980) Personal Communication-Seminar at New York Hospital Cornell-Weil- White Plains, NY Medical Center).

11 This interaction provides me with another opportunity to say that I typically do not initially know what a presenter's gratuitous comments mean; that said, in this vignette, I did know that the awkward placement of the word *currently* suggested an oddity that one sees in slips of the tongue and parapraxis; it was thus worth exploring. In *The Psychopathology of Everyday Life* (1901) and *Jokes and Their Relation to the Unconscious* (1905), Freud extended his understanding of the unconscious mind. He did so use the insights that he had gained from the psychoanalysis of neurotic patients. Starting with the observation that neurosis is an unconscious defense against intolerable experience, Freud now looked at a variety of so-called normal phenomena, such as slips of the tongue, which had previously been thought to be accidental, and jokes, where he demonstrated that joke telling, like dreaming, neurotic symptoms, and *Freudian slips*, all follow an orderly process where there is a release, or a blocking (repression), of thoughts and emotion followed by a failure of the repression. However, in these phenomena, the failure of repression is temporary, and the interference with the person's functioning is minor and brief. As we have seen, as an extension of Freud (1905)/ Reich (1949)/Reik (1948)/Winnicott/Bion in my own work I have applied this way of understanding somewhat odd placements of sentences, words or phrases and add-ons to sentences in the belief that these unusual words and phrases or unusual placement of words and phrases can provide us with insights into preconscious processes in the presenter. And, further, this deeper understanding of the *presenter* will ultimately lead us to a deeper understanding of the case that is being presented. In other words, I look not only at what the presenter says but also what he/she does not say or what he or she says oddly.

12 The process that I am describing in this new circumstance is a very different process than when a presenter is unaware that they are distorting the clinical material because of some preconscious enactment; in that circumstance, the 'reality' of the presenter's hiding is often quite clear to everyone in the room except for the presenter. In the example

I am talking about here, the listeners/observers of the presentation might typically feel confused by the material but they would typically believe that this confusion has to do with the nature of the patient's problems as these problems are directly being presented by the clinician. In fact, the presenter may actually be distorting some of the material typically in some misplaced *loyalty* toward the patient, that is, by presenting the patient as less critical/less disturbed.

13 I have said throughout this book that I have no 'false modesty.' It is important to state that having no false modesty is not the same as being unaware of one's limitations. For example, here is one thing that I know about myself; I am particularly reactive to (triggered by) people who attempt to make me feel guilty/ashamed and responsible for the bad things that have happened to them. If I begin work with such a person, I am acutely aware of my vulnerability to this, and consequently, I need to assess whether or not we are a 'good it' for their therapy. (In my history, my parents often employed shaming and guilt inducement as parental techniques and my tolerance for this was low even when I was a child…it is now even lower.) In this regard, as I have been saying throughout this book, I am always curious about my own mental processes/and reactions as well as the processes of others (my patients/students/presenters), and in this way, I can often 'catch' myself falling into errors. And, as an extra protection, as I suggest to all clinicians, one should have at least *one friend* in the profession who you can count on to always tell you the truth even if this or that particular truth is painful. For me, my best source of truth is my wife-also a psychologist/psychoanalyst/teacher-and she is certainly never shy about telling me when I am being too co. And, as an extra protection, as I suggest to all clinicians, one should have at least *one friend* in the profession who you can count on to always tell you the truth-even if this or that truth is painful. For me, my best source of truth is my wife-also a psychologist/psychoanalyst/teacher-and she is certainly never shy about telling me when I am being too confident/arrogant/misguided and/or not curious enough.

14 I want to thank Pazia Miller for her permission to include this helpful interchange.

15 Levinson, E. *The Fallacy of Understanding* and *the Anatomy of Change* (2005). London: Routledge.

References

Alexander, F., & French, T. (1946) *Psychoanalytic Therapy*. New York: Ronald Press.

Barber, J. P., Muran, J. C., McCarthy, K. S., & Keefe, R. J. (2013) Research on psychodynamic therapies. In M. J. Lambert (Ed.), *Bergin and Garfield's Handbook of Psychotherapy and Behavior, Change* (6th Ed., pp. 443–494). New York: John Wiley & Sons.Bion, W. R. (1961) *Experiences in Groups*. London: Tavistock Publications.

Bion, W. R. (1967) *Second Thoughts*. London: William Heinemann [Reprinted London: Karnac Books 1984].

Bion, W. R. (1976) Personal Communication.

Clark, K. B., & Clark, M. P. (1958) Racial identification and preference among Negro children. In E. L. Hartley (Ed.), *Readings in Social Psychology* (pp. 138–150). New York: Holt, Rinehart, and Winston.

Festinger, L. (1957). *A Theory of Cognitive Dissonance*. California: Stanford University Press.

Frawley-O'Dea, M. G. (1997) Who's doing what to whom?' Supervision and sexual abuse. *Contemporary Psychoanalysis, 33*(1), 5–18.

Freud, S. (1901) The psychopathology of everyday life. In *The Standard Edition of the Complete Psychological Works of Sigmund Freud, Volume VI* (pp. vii–296). London: Hogarth Press.

Freud, S. (1905) Jokes and their relation to the unconscious. In *The Standard Edition of the Complete Psychological Works of Sigmund Freud, Volume VIII* (pp. 1–247). London: Hogarth Press.

Freud, S. (1912) Recommendations to physicians practising psycho-analysis. In *The Standard Edition of the Complete Psychological Works of Sigmund Freud, Volume XII* (pp. 109–120). London: Hogarth Press.Haley, J. (1963) *Strategies of Psychotherapy*. New York: Grune & Stratton.

Kernberg, O. (1980) *Personal Communication* Seminar at Weil Cornell New York Hospital-White Plains, N Y Medical Center; sponsored by the Postdoctoral Program in Group Psychotherapy, Adelphi University, Adelphi University, Garden City, New York.

Kernberg, O. F., Michael A. S., Harold W. K., Carr, A. C., & Appelbaum, A. H. (1989) *Psychodynamic Psychotherapy of Borderline Patients*. New York: Basic Books.

Levenson, E. (2005) *The Fallacy of Understanding* and *The Anatomy of Change*. London: Routledge.Mendelsohn, R. (1978) Critical factors in short-term psychotherapy: A summary. *Bulletin of the Menninger Clinic, 42*, 133–148 (This article includes a case supervised by W.R. Bion in 1976).

Mendelsohn, R. (2022) *Freudian Thought for the Contemporary Clinician*. London: Routledge.

Mendelsohn, R., & Harmatz, M. (1977) Length of Stay and behavior patterns of hospitalized schizophrenic patients. *Psychiatric Services, 28*(4), 273–277.

Miller, C. H., & Hedges, D. W. (2008) Scrupulosity disorder: An overview and introductory analysis. *Journal of Anxiety Disorders, 22*(6), 1042–1045.Reik, T. (1932/1959) The unknown murderer. In J. Farrar (Ed.), *The Compulsion to Confess and the Need for Punishment* (pp. 3–173). New York: Farrar, Straus, and Cudahy.

Reik, T. (1948) *Listening with the Third Ear*. New York: Grove Press.Stern, D. (2005) In E. Levenson (Ed.), *The Fallacy of Understanding* and *The Anatomy of Change*. London: Routledge.

Chapter 7

Conclusion—Creating a Space for the *'Magic'* to Occur/ Teaching the *'Magic'* to Others

As I have said from the beginning, this is a book that is about more than how to do Case Formulation. My goal has been to present a comprehensive method of formulating the psychotherapy case, as well as teaching my new method of case formulation to others.

To do this, I began by tracing the first work done on the formulation of the therapeutic treatment plan in psychodynamic psychotherapy. Theories that have included the formulation of a full plan for a treatment, from the initial patient contact(s) through the working phase of the therapy to its conclusion, were reviewed; this included the early works of Freud (1901, 1905) Reich (1949) Reik (1948), Menninger (1958), Bion (1962) and Winnicott (1949, 1973) as well as some more recent works (Billow and Mendelsohn 1990) that look at the complex transference/countertransference and patient/therapist interactions.

Following this, I presented my own approach to case formulation, an approach that I have been developing since I began my doctoral studies in clinical psychology more than 50 years ago. This training and experience have focused on devising new methods of treatment, of case formulation, of case supervision, of treatment planning, and of case conceptualization.

In the next part of this book, I demonstrated the ways in which my approach differs from traditional clinical supervision, as well as from the typical presentation of clinical material by a student in the case, seminar setting. I also showed why and how I believe that my approach is more helpful and effective in very quickly organizing and directing the complex data of the 'clinical encounter,' from the very beginning of the therapy to its conclusion.

As I have continuously said, I believe that clinicians learn about their patients in a variety of ways and that they both experience and even *understand* each patient on both conscious and preconscious levels. As you have seen, my students' (and some of my colleague's) understanding of my Case Consultation work is that it an example of a kind of *clinical magic*. However, as I have also said throughout this book, there is a much less glamorous explanation to my skill in case consultation, an explanation that makes my approach considerably more accessible to all clinicians. My approach concerns the identification by the Consultant to the Presenter of preconscious information that the Presenter

DOI: 10.4324/9781003375944-8

in fact already possesses somewhere inside of himself/herself! Thus, as we have seen over and over again, I discourage the labeling of the patient's *presenting problem(s)* at the beginning of a case presentation so as to not lead us astray with the patient's (and often with the Presenter's) current, often somewhat limited, understanding of the problem, and also so that I/we can focus on a precon-scious, as well as a conscious, understanding of each case, an understanding that I believe the presenting clinician typically *actually already knows* somewhere inside of himself/herself—even though he/she may not know that they know it or that they knew it once and they later *forgot* it (i.e., what was once conscious has now become preconscious)!

That said, ironically, over the many years that I have been doing Case Consultations in this way, even with Presenters that have some knowledge about *what I do* and *how I do it,* many still want to experience my approach as a kind of 'magic.' I have detailed some of the reasons why I believe this to be so as well as what I do in my efforts to dispel this notion.

What appears to some to be magical insights into clinical cases is in fact a series of steps that includes a detailed/standard inquiry during the Clinical Presentation. Throughout the presentation experience, I continually point out that I never have a totally clear, accurate, or definitive understanding of what the Presenter's *precon-scious* comments fully mean (these comments are what I have, tongue-in-cheek, called the Presenter's *gratuitous remarks*). I emphasize that what I do have is only a beginning, often preconscious, recognition that the Presenter's remarks mean *something.* That is, the Presenter's remarks alert me to the psychological fact that his/her comments mean *something more* than a conscious/ factual understanding about the following:

1 This Presenter;
2 the patient to be presented;
3 their mix/relationship; and
4 the very act of this Presenter presenting this person to this group at this particu-lar period.

The process of unraveling the psychological meaning of all of this and of putting that meaning in the context of a valuable learning experience (a learning process that includes a viable psychological theory of motivation and etiology, a technique of treatment, a theory of technique, and the formulation of a preliminary treatment plan for the case) is what I have attempted to teach each of you in this book. I did so by describing a theory of clinical communication that includes both the manifest content and the latent content of patient/therapist and teacher-Consultant/Presenter interactions. I further highlighted my points by including several vignettes, from my many years of being a practicing clinician, a teacher of clinical process, a clini-cal supervisor, and a clinical consultant.[1]

I also want to state my belief that those students/clinicians and colleagues who have parodied me over the many years that I have teaching and training clinicians are in fact accurate about one thing, I am both a very accomplished clinician/ therapist/ supervisor/ consultant and, more to the point, *I am not afraid to make educated guesses in the quest to more deeply understand and make meaning out of what is occurring in a therapy.* How did I become this?

To answer this question, I have looked deeply into the work of those who study expertise.

Schulman (1982; also in Mendelsohn 2022) suggests that writers in psychoanalysis and, I would add, writers working to understand all the dynamic psychotherapies have not successfully incorporated a shift in the epistemology of psychoanalytic science into their approaches to depth psychological understanding. Scientific knowledge in many fields where interpretation plays an important role is not dependent on controlled studies, but rather upon the care with which multiple and redundant checks are applied as work proceeds. The psychotherapy clinician recognizes how this error checking process is so much a part of their daily work.

Do experienced psychotherapists have a special kind of expertise? Studies of expertise in many fields have shown the most important difference between experts and individuals who are less successful in their fields is *their extensive detailed knowledge,* which permits them to focus on problem solution rather than following a set method. Problem-solving strategies employed by such experts tend to be carried out with considerable flexibility.

The experts don't use cognitive methods identifiably different from those used by others; rather, they demonstrate what Schulman has called a 'well-stocked mind.' Yet, it is rare that the exact nature of the expertise can be stated in many fields, as in psychodynamic psychotherapy. The clinical situation, where the clinician has an extensive and wide exposure to the life and mind of each patient, constitutes a very special form of expertise about each patient that can be underestimated and has not been studied carefully.

To summarize, and to expand upon what you have heard up to this point, below is the formula for my *magic.* Further, I would add that by following the concepts that are presented below, and that I have discussed throughout this book, in their functional relationship to each other, one can arrive at a detailed understanding of the major clinical issues of each presented case, as well as an understanding of what to do, and when to do it, in any psychodynamic therapy. I recognize that I am promising a lot.

I have proposed that in all clinical encounters, the following processes occur:

1 Along with the conscious processing of thoughts, feelings, and actions, there is also an inducement of preconscious thoughts, feelings, and actions. (And, in this scenario, most typically any *pressure toward action or pull toward feelings in the clinician* occurs in a kind of *inducement* process called an *enactment.*)
2 All these inducements and enactments produce transference and countertransference reactions in each of the parties (patient(s), therapist-Presenter, and supervisor/teacher/Consultant).

3 These transference/countertransference reactions are the result of both identification and projective identification.
4 All reactions in both parties in the teacher/student relationship (therapist/ Presenter and teacher/Consultant-observer) that are typically labeled as countertransference can also be understood to be parallel processes in that each of the parties is *inducing reactions in the other.*

Following the steps described above will allow any clinician to decode all of the preconscious transactions that are occurring. Once these preconscious messages are decoded, the messages can be used to reconstruct, at the deepest levels of meaning, everything that is occurring in the clinical encounter. This is the so-called magic that I have referred to throughout this book, nothing less/nothing more. Thus, as can be noted in the many examples that I have presented throughout this book, when one listens closely to a Presenter's case material, without any preconceived notions that might have arisen from hearing a *prepackaged presenting problem and current history of the treatment,* what emerges are clues that can lead the Consultant to a fresh perspective about the clinical material. And, ironically, this fresh perspective had in fact already been present in the mind of the Presenting clinician all along, but for one reason or another, it had been *...lost in translation...* at some earlier time in the history of the therapy.

I have suggested that, while for some readers the above terms (such as projective identification and/or preconscious transactions) may be new and cumbersome, once they are used a few times and then mastered, the rest is simply about listening closely for the appearance of these functions and correlating them to each other. In this regard, what I have offered in my model is not so different from the way that Freud (1905, 1909, 1912, 1918), Reik (1948, 1959), Bion (1962) and Winnicott (1973) each did their clinical work. That is, each of these clinicians/theorists *reconstructed* a patient's conflictual history from his/her symptoms/current conflicts and contiguously *constructed meaning* from the day residue, free associations from the patient's dreams, and all other associations that occurred in the therapy.

Creating a Space for 'the Magic' to Occur and Teaching 'the Magic' to Others

How does a clinician allow for a *space* between not becoming an arrogant 'know-it-all' (and thereby losing one's curiosity), while, at the same time, allowing oneself to possess expertise that some might perceive as *magical*? I will now attempt to answer this question.

To review, I began this book by asking "Why would I want to write another book about psychodynamic case formulation?"

I also noted that there are already several very good books available and some particularly good books about a related topic: clinical supervision.

That said, for many years (Mendelsohn 2017) I have been exploring how to teach psychodynamic case formulation as an area of *expertise that can be practiced, taught, and learned.* In this regard, I have struggled with a related issue: how does a teacher avoid the seduction of believing in his/her own omnipotence, while at the same time being open and able to allow himself/herself to recognize their role as an effective teacher/supervisor/Consultant?

An effective teacher/Consultant *possesses expertise, communicates this expertise clearly, and teaches this expertise to others.* Throughout this book I have attempted to demonstrate that one can practice and teach the so-called magic, that is, recognize that this expertise might temporarily afford them a special ability. This is the ability to be the only person in the room who is currently able to observe and translate the preconscious transactions that are occurring in a clinical encounter and to reconstruct those transactions to present, at the least, a rudimentary understanding of the 'case.' If one is also able to place the expertise in a space where one recognizes their 'special abilities' but also knows that these skills are teachable (and thus they are not at all magical), then the *expert* is also the *teacher.* And, additionally, the magic is what we can teach, and it is what others can learn; it is an expertise that comes from a series of functionally related processes that are teachable/learnable.

So, given my reputation as a legend and as a weaver of magic spells (as well as whatever 'magic' I have presented to you in this book), the reader might ask the following question—have I succeeded in performing my task of demystifying and teaching you my so-called magical skills?

Here is my answer: I think that I did, if we can agree that the so-called magic that I have shown the reader is not magic at all, but that it is the elucidation of a number of principles regarding conscious/preconscious and unconscious communication processes—processes that were eluded to and even discussed by psychoanalytic writers from Freud to Reich to Reik to Winnicott and Bion, and to Menninger and Billow & Mendelsohn.

However, I do believe that the processes you have seen throughout this book are very powerful. They can be taught, and particularly for newer clinicians, these techniques and, in particular, the ways of thinking connected to them will be extremely helpful in decoding the meaning of each clinical interaction, communicating that meaning in a helpful way to one's patients, and this will result in helping to alter the symptoms and character issues of the patient. This training will also prepare one to become an expert clinician and an expert supervisor/teacher. I recognize that I am promising a lot.

To illustrate again my thinking about how to create a space for 'magic' to occur, I will now quote an anecdote from my recent book *Freudian Thought for the Contemporary Reader* (2022, p. 87) about the sudden appearance of an early memory:

"In a recent class, an old memory (of mine) suddenly came back to me:

I recently had an experience in a Group Therapy Session for a group that I currently lead; this memory made me think again about the creative power of the unconscious/preconscious.

Here is the context, and then the memory: During a group session last week, a memory returned to me that I hadn't thought about in many years. It was so wonderful because it's so obvious when you hear about it. The context is that in the group, there are two male group members who were talking about an old conflict in the group between the two of them, which I naively thought had been resolved. And, I said something about the 'resolution.' However, the next thing I knew, both were enraged (at first, at each other, then at the group, and then…finally, at me). They were both threatening to quit the group, even threatening physical violence against each other. Given each man's history and psychological dynamics, physical violence against the other…while not impossible…would be quite unlikely.

Here's the memory:

…I'm about three/four years old and my mother is talking to a neighbor on the first floor of our apartment building (in the NYC Borough of Queens). We are at the top of a long flight of stairs that lead down (many) steps to the basement, which has an open door because the basement is where the washers and the dryers are- to clean the tenants' clothes. I am sitting on my tricycle, perched at the very edge of the stairway (I believe that my mother was just about to take me outside to ride…but this could be a *secondary elaboration…* remember that term from *The Interpretation of Dreams*)? I see nothing else in this memory, although the story that I was told later was that the superintendent of the building who was in that basement at that time- saw me flying down the stairs, and he witnessed helplessly as I smacked-face first- into a basement wall, breaking my nose in three places…

I hadn't had this memory in a very long time, but it came back to me when I was thinking about this class and about what had happened in the therapy group. Early memories come back to us at various times in our lives (in the telling of this I am now 79 years old), and it is as if the unconscious wants to remind us of something, teach us something. Maybe I had been feeling too arrogant, a little too brass, or rash, or reckless in the group, *or even in this class*. In that case, the memory would serve as a *warning…* stop flying around…get back to earth. Perhaps, it also says something about my mother's care or her inattention, and it is a reminder to me: *Don't be as inattentive as she was on that day.* This point comes home as I now have two young grandchildren and I am reminded again about how much attention a young child requires to protect the child from danger. Thus, this might also be a *rebuff* against myself: you did not protect these group members from themselves and protect the group from the anger in the room…as expressed by these two group members. That is, by being *inattentive, preoccupied, perhaps too interested in some other conversations, you failed in your protective function….*

Perhaps this is a good time to emphasize, again, what I have said throughout this book; that in my *magic*, I am following and extending Freud (and his followers) in my approach, because I rely on the technique of reconstruction to base each of my hypotheses. Freud answered criticisms of reconstruction by explaining that the veracity of the reconstructed event is secondary to the meaning co-constructed by the patient and the psychoanalyst. Freud's defense of reconstruction was that the specific details of the experience might be less important than the outcome of the process. Engaging in the reconstruction demonstrates interest and willingness to cooperate with the patient, conveys hope that seemingly disorienting or difficult to understand content can be understood and worked through, and bolsters the alliance between the patient and the clinician. In this regard, it helps to recognize that it is okay to offer several reconstructions or interpretations and that each may be not quite right. A process of revision and cooperation is likely what leads to making valuable discoveries about a patient's preconscious and unconscious processes. Second, reconstruction may be advantageous because it is not concerned with the actual events but instead allows for an understanding of the past to evolve with the patient, their level of insight, and the changes that are occurring both inside and outside of their awareness. In sum, from Freud we have learned that reconstruction is particularly useful when we remember that all interpretations are tentative, more related to co-created meaning than 'objective truth'; this helps to make us more flexible about both change and revision.

It follows, then, that it is best if the clinician works to create a *space* for his/her own history, training, and clinical experience so that all of it can help us to see both where we *get it right* as well as *where our history and experiences might be a hindrance to understanding our cases.*

A Further Word about '*Teacher Omnipotence*' and the Vignettes

As I did frequently throughout this book, I now want to say a bit more about the complex issues going on within the *expert*. On the one hand, the expert must struggle with not denying the special skills and power of a supervisor/teacher/Consultant—yet, at the same time, he/she must learn how to not encourage students' fantasies of omnipotence. Thus, in this book, I've worked hard to teach each of you new ways to look closely at the supervisees' fantasy of 'supervisor omnipotence' (*the so-called magic*) parodied in the 'skit' presented at the beginning of this book. Let's look at this fantasy more closely now:

I suggest that omnipotent fantasies about the clinician/teacher are often not discouraged by their students and that these same students may even subtly encourage such fantasies (sometimes the supervisor encourages them, as well). At some level, beginning clinicians are hoping that their teacher/supervisor has all of the truth/all the answers—that is, all the *magic* to teach them as clinical work can be both quite confusing and somewhat scary. And, of course, sometimes the supervisor will also feel this, perhaps for similar reasons. However, one thing I hope that I have to communicate to you throughout this work is the following: if the supervisor/teacher can begin to recognize and understand the pushes and pulls inside of himself or herself to be omnipotent and the seductive pushes and pulls that are also coming from one's patients as well as from one's students, this will allow each of us to *create a space between all of the pressures within us* that can be *held* alongside of our rational desire to utilize our well-stocked mind, that is, to utilize and not deny one's expertise! What we will then have instead is a well-earned expertise, living side by side, with one's humility, fallibility, curiosity and with one's awe about the mystery of the human condition.

Further, I propose that the best way to accomplish all that I have offered above is to present a comprehensive model of how the clinician/teacher/Consultant thinks clearly and cogently about his/her cases and how he/she thinks about the best ways to perform our work. In other words, the why and how we make the choices and decisions that we make, the why and how we ask the questions that we ask, and the why and how we come to the formulations that we come up with. Reality has a way of making *magic* seem *less magical.*

To summarize:

This book has presented a revised model of psychodynamic case formulation that encourages exploring the preconscious transactions as well as the dynamics of the Presenter/Consultant from the exact moment of initial presentation (including the first few words spoken) about the 'case'. Why even those first few moments? I hope that this book has explained that, as well.

Examples of my case formulation process came from many hours of supervision over five years (2018, 2019, 2020, 2021, and 2022). The examples/excerpts of actual clinical presentations were recorded, transcribed, edited, and then integrated so that they maintain a sequence and rhythm. They were included to demonstrate that while the parody of an 'example' of my supervisory work in *the skit* presented at the beginning of this book is silly and exaggerated, like many parodies, there is a certain grain of truth in this example in that, while what I do might sometimes appear to seem like magic, what is occurring is that as the Teacher/Consultant I am simply following all of the threads of the therapist/Presenter as he/she presents their actual clinical interaction in the session to be understood. In this regard, in all of the examples presented in this book, the identity of both the therapist/Presenter and the patient (or patient(s) the couple, family, or therapy group) has been disguised, and the data about all members of this clinical encounter (except for me) have been altered to preserve anonymity, while not altering the essential elements of the dynamics, defensive structure, transference-countertransference, unconscious object relations, and preconscious transactions of the experience.

I hope that I have shed some light on how one can teach *magic* and how one can demonstrate the 'it' of psychodynamic consultation so that it is recognized to be both 'not magical' and, actually, quite doable.

Formulating a Therapeutic Plan: A Final Summary

Even those psychoanalytic therapists who treat patients more frequently than once per week, so that there is a considerable amount of time and clinical material available to draw conclusions, now recognize that one must formulate a plan for the treatment very early on in the sessions. While this plan is always going to be flexible and altered with new information, as Reich (1933) reminds us, it is best to have some general schema as opposed to following the patient wherever he or she may lead us.

Yet, all patients who enter therapy are not the same: Even with neurotic patients, one must be sensitive to closeness and silence with someone who is on the neurotic end but has Schizoid dynamics; one needs to be alerted to affect with an Obsessive-Compulsive patient; one needs to be particularly careful with boundary issues and triangulation concerns when working with patients with hysterical features.

So, *what* is *Formulating a Therapeutic Plan?* Is it simply a general outline like what I just described above?

Yes, but it is also more than this; it is generating a series of dynamic hypotheses, having them tested, confirmed, and disconfirmed, until a reasonable and coherent understanding of the person's dynamic issues and key incidents in his/her life that have triggered current symptoms/affects and conflicts are both understood and mastered with talk therapy.

With this formula in mind, we can divide any psychotherapy treatment into two phases:

1   A dynamic formulation: that is, what triggered the current conflict(s) and what are its roots in the person's history?
2   The treatment itself: this includes both a working through of the above conflicts, followed by a termination phase of the therapy.

From Menninger (1958) and Alexander & French (1946), we have learned what distinguishes a psychodynamic therapist; there are two features: (1) being free of the desire to instantly cure and (2) recognizing that everything that the patient and the therapist does has meaning. We have also seen that at an initial clinical meeting, the therapist often knows a lot about the patient that, over time and with more therapy/patients details, the therapist begins to forget. That is, over time it is not uncommon for a clinician to lose one's perspective.

From Freud (1901, 1905), we have learned so much, but particularly for our purposes, the importance of the *process of reconstruction* in connecting current communication (manifest and latent) to its historical antecedents.

From W. Reich (1948), we have seen an emphasis not only on what patient *does and says* but also on what *is not done and not said*; these are what Reich calls the latent resistances.

T. Reik's (1959) observations suggest that humans have a deep need to communicate our deepest parts to others. Further, this observation lends support to my own theory of preconscious communication.

Winnicott (1973) considered that the "mother's technique of holding, of bathing, of feeding, everything she did for the baby, added up to the child's first idea of the mother", as well as fostering the ability to experience the body as the place where one securely lives. This led to the idea of a therapeutic 'holding environment,' an idea expanded upon by Bion.

Bion's (1962) concept of the mother or therapist, who in her reverie and via her alpha functioning[3] transmits to the acutely distressed baby or patient the seeds of the capacity to think rather than to evacuate, is in some ways like Winnicott's 'holding', although Winnicott's concept seems to involve a less active and perhaps less intrusive process on the part of the mother, but one that is very protective of the child's fragile ego.

In the late 1980s and into the 1990s, my colleague (Dr. Richard Billow) and I began to explore the complex processes of transference and countertransference that occur early in a therapy, even in the early minutes of an initial interview.

And, finally, other non-psychodynamic clinicians (Haley 1963, 1973; Erickson 1964) have taught us again the power of language to influence/communicate/ obscure/control/imply and to create meaning in others at both the conscious and the preconscious levels.

Summary of This Last Chapter

In this book, I traced the early work done on the formulation of the therapeutic treatment plan in psychodynamic psychotherapy. I reviewed theories that include the formulation of the treatment plan from the initial patient contact(s) to the working phase of the therapy, such as the early work of Freud (1918), Reich (1949), Reik (1948), Bion (1962), and Winnicott (1973) as well as more recent works (Billow and Mendelsohn 1990) which look at the complex transference/counter-transference patient/therapist interactions. Following this, I presented my own current approach to case formulation and demonstrated how it differs from ongoing clinical supervision. I also suggested that my approach is very helpful and effective in organizing, as well as directing, the complex data of the clinical encounter from the very beginning of the therapy to a successful conclusion.

To demonstrate what I have said, I presented many examples, both of student presentations of clinical cases and examples of my own therapy. An important goal was to demonstrate that the so-called magic that my students' (see above—the *Preface* of this book) parodied about me is not magic at all. It is the simple translation of latent content to its underlying manifest content (i.e., translating manifest to latent from therapist to patient and from consultant to Presenter).

As I said throughout this book, at the beginning of any clinical interaction, I don't necessarily have a clear or accurate understanding of the deeper (preconscious) meaning of any patient or any student/Presenter's comments, only a beginning understanding that these remarks mean *something*. That is, the Presenter's remarks typically alert me to the psychological fact that their comments mean *something available but as yet unverbalized* about the following:

1 This presenter,
2 the patient that is currently being presented,
3 their mix/relationship, and
4 the very act of this Presenter presenting this person to this group at this period.

The process of unraveling the psychological meaning of all of this and of putting this meaning in the context of a valuable learning experience (a learning process that includes a viable psychological theory of motivation and etiology, a technique, a theory of technique, and even the formulation of a preliminary treatment plan for the case) is what I have worked hard to teach each of you in this book. I did so by describing a theory of clinical communication that includes both the manifest and latent content of patient/therapist and teacher/Presenter interactions, and I highlighted my points by including many vignettes from my many years of being a practicing clinician, a teacher of clinical process, and a clinical supervisor.

Finally, it is important to state one bit of irony in my novel approach. That is, after I have achieved some (often profound) understanding via a decoding of the preconscious enactments of both the therapist and the patient (and sometimes also of the clinical supervisor) what I have uncovered about the patient is simply this: (1) the correlation between this person's presenting complaints and his/her current behavior with (2) his/her traumatic history and development. Yet, often I have learned nothing more than this. The person's values/likes and dislikes/taste and sense of aliveness/deadness in processing their world often remain unknown to me. Thus, while I now know quite a bit, including some very important things about them, I do not know everything. This *other* understanding can only come from the long-term unfolding of the person and their *essence* in later sessions with their therapist.

Final Words

Throughout this book, I have suggested that preconscious processes such as enactments, inducements, and projective identification are ubiquitous in all human interaction *and that they are not always pathological*. I have also presented reasons as to why it might be tempting for students and other clinicians to view any special examples of clinical expertise as a kind of *magic*. However, I have worked hard to argue against this temptation. I have demonstrated that if one follows the preconscious threads in any clinical encounter and correlates these threads with all extant data, the clinician can arrive at a place where he/she can make meaning out of every clinical experience. That is, by following a clear set of principles, one can make meaning where there was no meaning before. This is my *clinical magic*, nothing less and nothing more.

Note

1 The translation of a metaphor is one way to understand and decode the hidden (precon-scious) meaning of an enactment; that is, the meaning of an act or behavior out of the patient's awareness, that occurs in a therapy—typically as an attempt by the patient to work through this person's traumatic childhood. We have seen many such enactments and their translations throughout this book.

References

Alexander, F., & French, T. (1946) *Psychoanalytic Therapy*. New York: Ronald Press.

Billow, R., & Mendelsohn, R. (1990) The interviewer's presenting problems in the initial interview. *Bulletin of the Menninger Clinic, 54*(3), 391–400.

Bion, W. (1962) *Learning from Experience*. London: Heineman.

Erickson, M. (1964) An hypnotic technique for resistant patients. *Journal of the American Society for Clinical Hypnosis, VII*(1), 8–33.

Freud, S. (1901) The psychopathology of everyday life. In *The Standard Edition of the Complete Psychological Works of Sigmund Freud, Volume VI* (pp. vii–296). London: Hogarth Press.

Freud, S. (1909) Notes upon a case of obsessional neurosis. In *The Standard Edition of the Complete Psychological Works of Sigmund Freud, Volume X* (pp. 151–318): Two Case Histories ('Little Hans' and the 'Rat Man'). London: Hogarth Press.

Freud, S. (1912) Recommendations to physicians practising psycho-analysis. In *The Standard Edition of the Complete Psychological Works of Sigmund Freud, Volume XII* (pp. 109–120). London: Hogarth Press.

Freud, S. (1918) From the history of an infantile neurosis. In *The Standard Edition of the Complete Psychological Works of Sigmund Freud, Volume XVII* (pp. 7–122). London: Hogarth Press.

Freud, S. (1905) Jokes and their relation to the unconscious. In *The Standard Edition of the Complete Psychological Works of Sigmund Freud, Volume VIII* (pp. 1–247). London: Hogarth Press.

Haley, J. (1963) *Strategies of Psychotherapy*. New York: Grune & Stratton.

Haley, J. (1973) *Uncommon Therapy: The Psychiatric Techniques of Milton H. Erickson, M.D.* New York: W.W. Norton.

Mendelsohn, R. (2017) *A Three factor Model of Couples Therapy*. Lanham, MD: Lexington Books/Rowman & Littlefield.

Mendelsohn, R (2022) *Freudian Thought for the Contemporary Reader*. London: Routledge.

Menninger, K. (1958) *Theory of Psychoanalytic Technique*. New York: Basic Books.

Reich, W. (1933) *Character Analysis*. New York: Simon and Schuster.

Reich, W. (1949) *Character Analysis*. New York: Noonday Press.

Reid, T. (1948) *Listening with the third ear*. New York: Farrar, Strauss.

Reik, T. (1959) The compulsion to confess. In J. Farrar (Ed.), *The Compulsion to Confess and the Need for Punishment* (pp. 176–356). New York: Farrar, Straus, and Cudahy (Original work published 1925).

Shulman, M. A. (1982) Piagetian developmental psychology. *Psychoanalytic Review, 69*(3), 411–414.

Winnicott, D. W. (1973) *The Child, the Family, and the Outside World* (p. 17 and p. 44). London: Middlesex.

Winnicott, D. W. (1949) Hate in the countertransference. *International Journal of Psychoanalysis 30*, 69–74.

Index

Note: Page numbers followed by "n" denote endnotes.

For Product Safety Concerns and Information please contact our EU
representative GPSR@taylorandfrancis.com
Taylor & Francis Verlag GmbH, Kaufingerstraße 24, 80331 München, Germany

www.ingramcontent.com/pod-product-compliance
Lightning Source LLC
Chambersburg PA
CBHW050657280326
41932CB00015B/2938